PICTURE BOOK OF
PSALMS

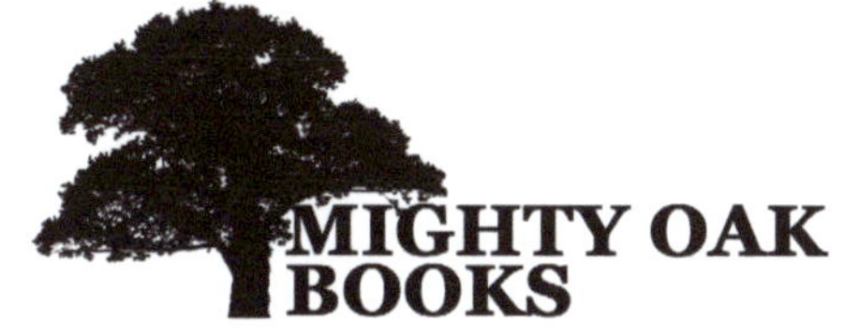

I will give thanks
to You, LORD,
with all my heart;
I will tell of all
Your wonderful
deeds.

Psalm 9:1

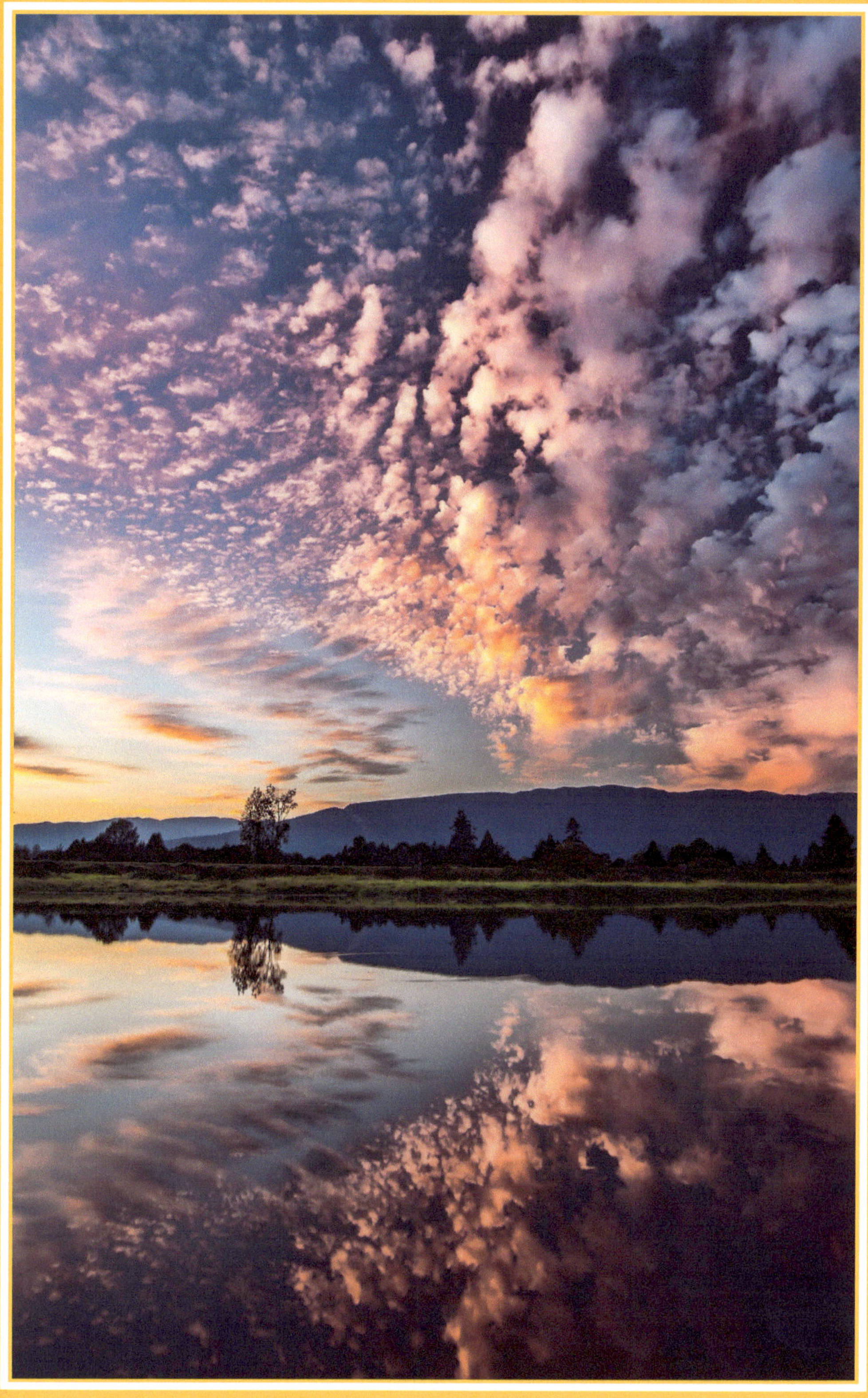

For with You is the fountain of life; in Your light we see light.

Psalm 36:9

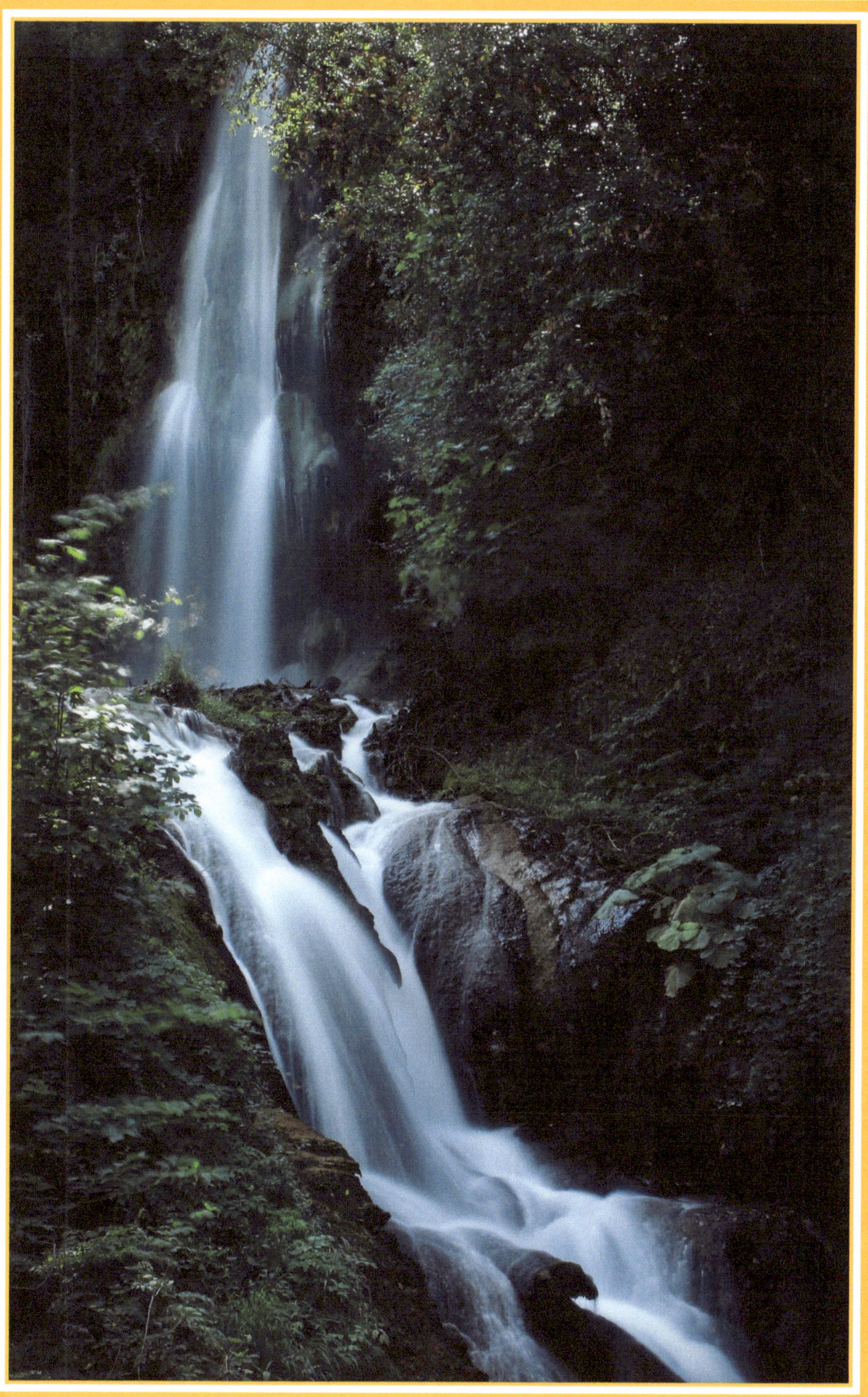

For great is Your love, reaching to the heavens; Your faithfulness reaches to the skies.

Psalm 57:10

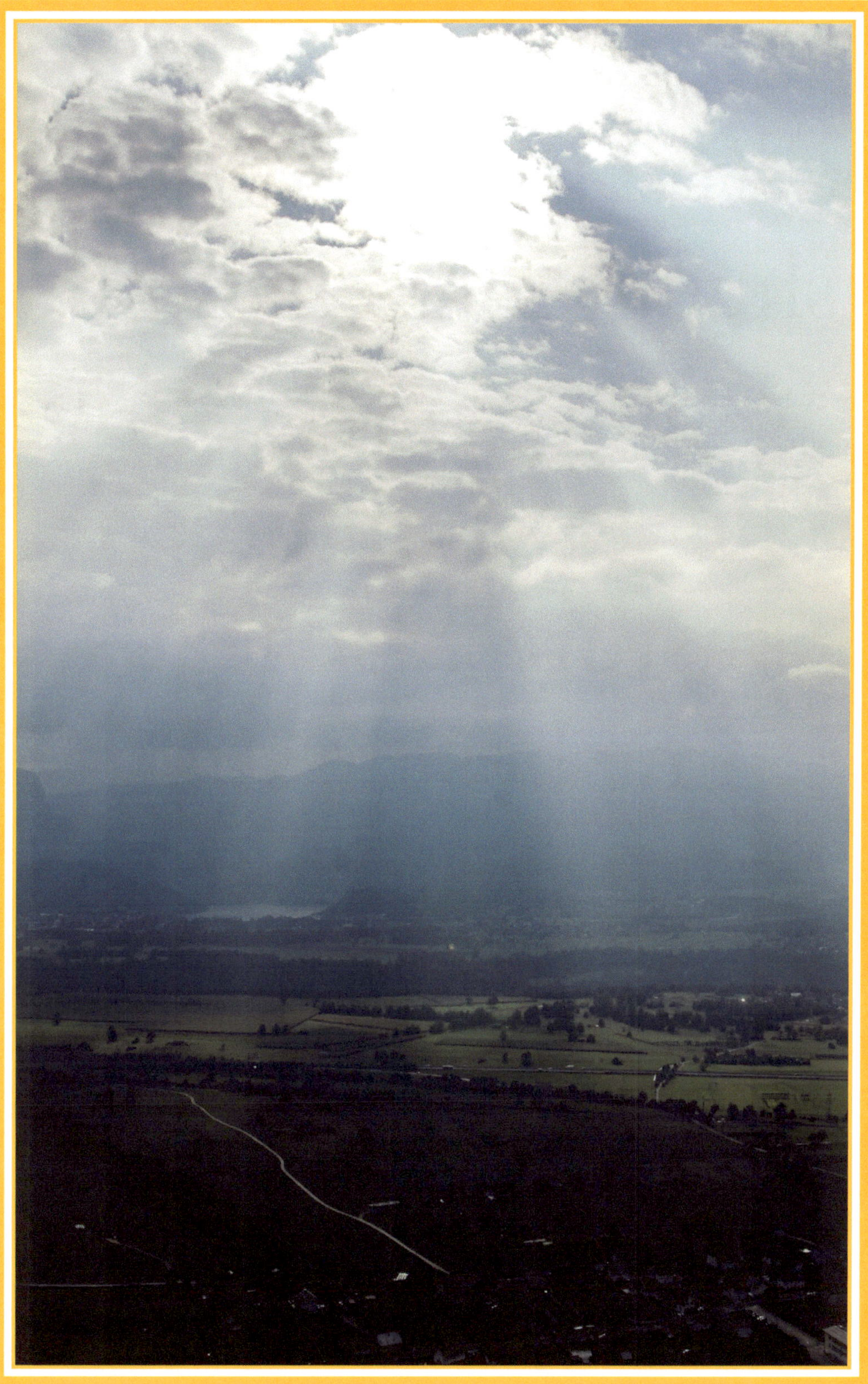

The LORD is my shepherd; I shall not want. He makes me lie down in green pastures. He leads me beside still waters. He restores my soul.

Psalm 23:1-3

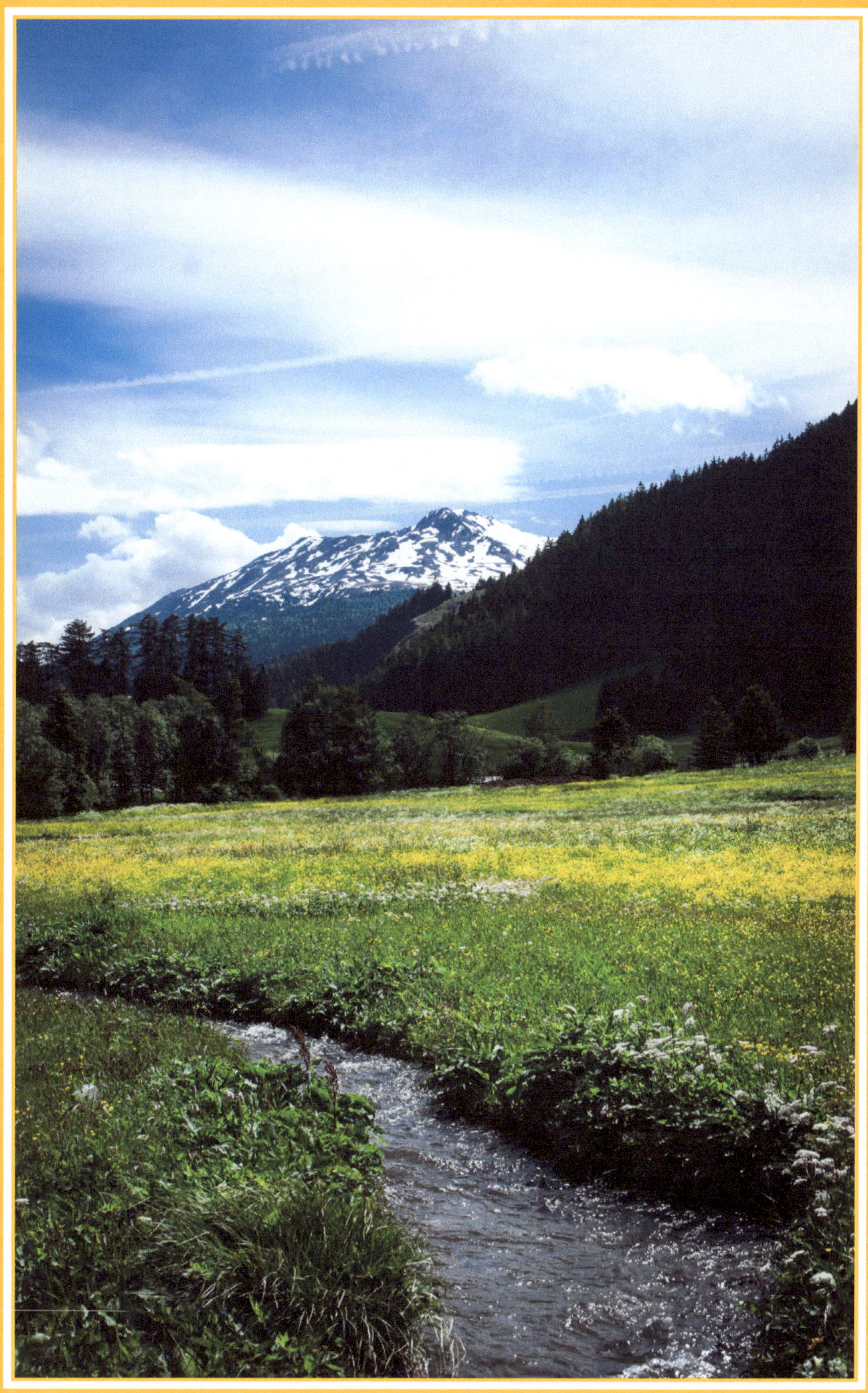

The LORD is my light and my salvation— whom shall I fear? The Lord is the stronghold of my life— of whom shall I be afraid?

Psalm 27:1

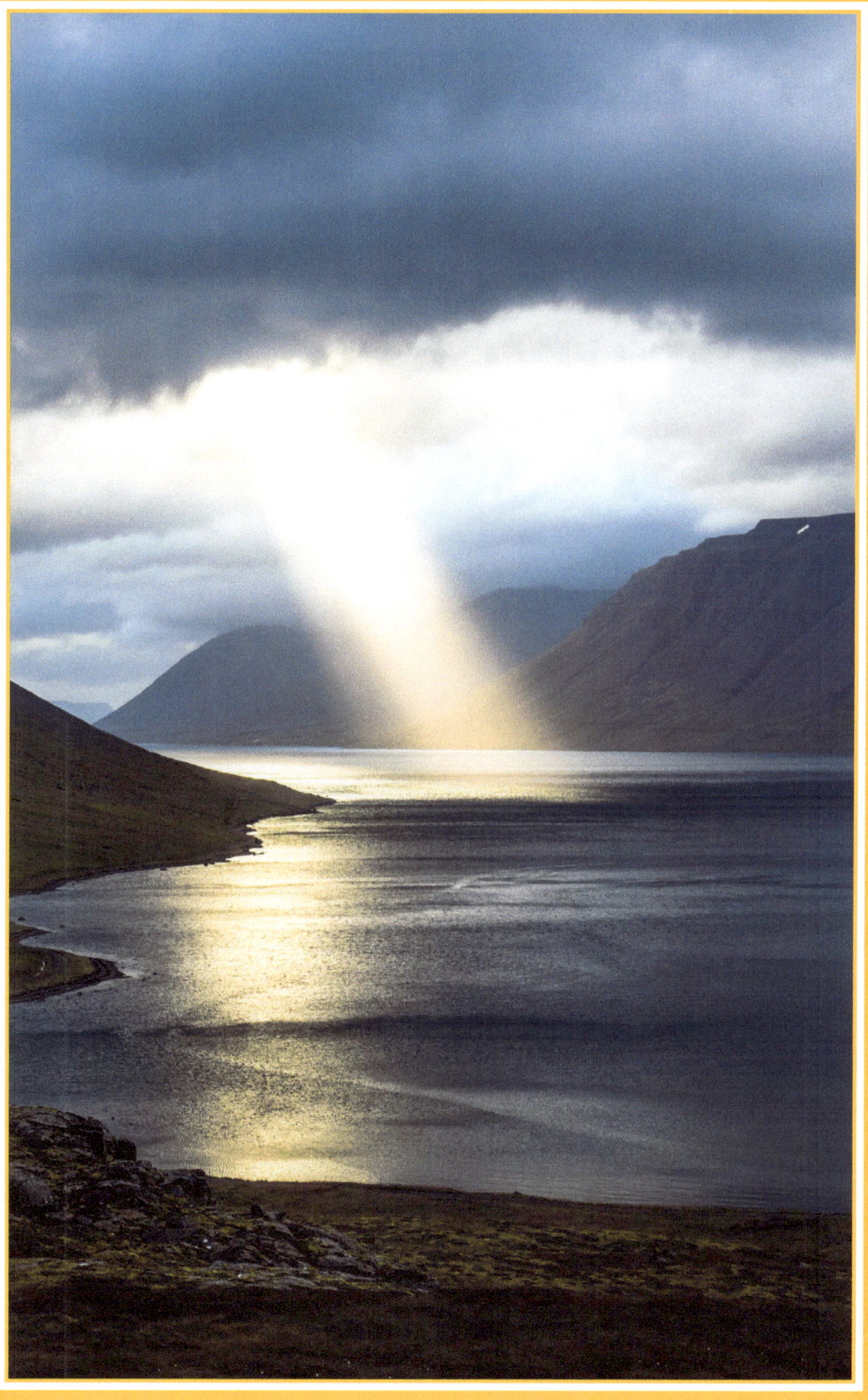

The LORD is my rock, my fortress and my savior; my God is my rock, in whom I find protection. He is my shield, the power that saves me, and my place of safety.

Psalms 18:2

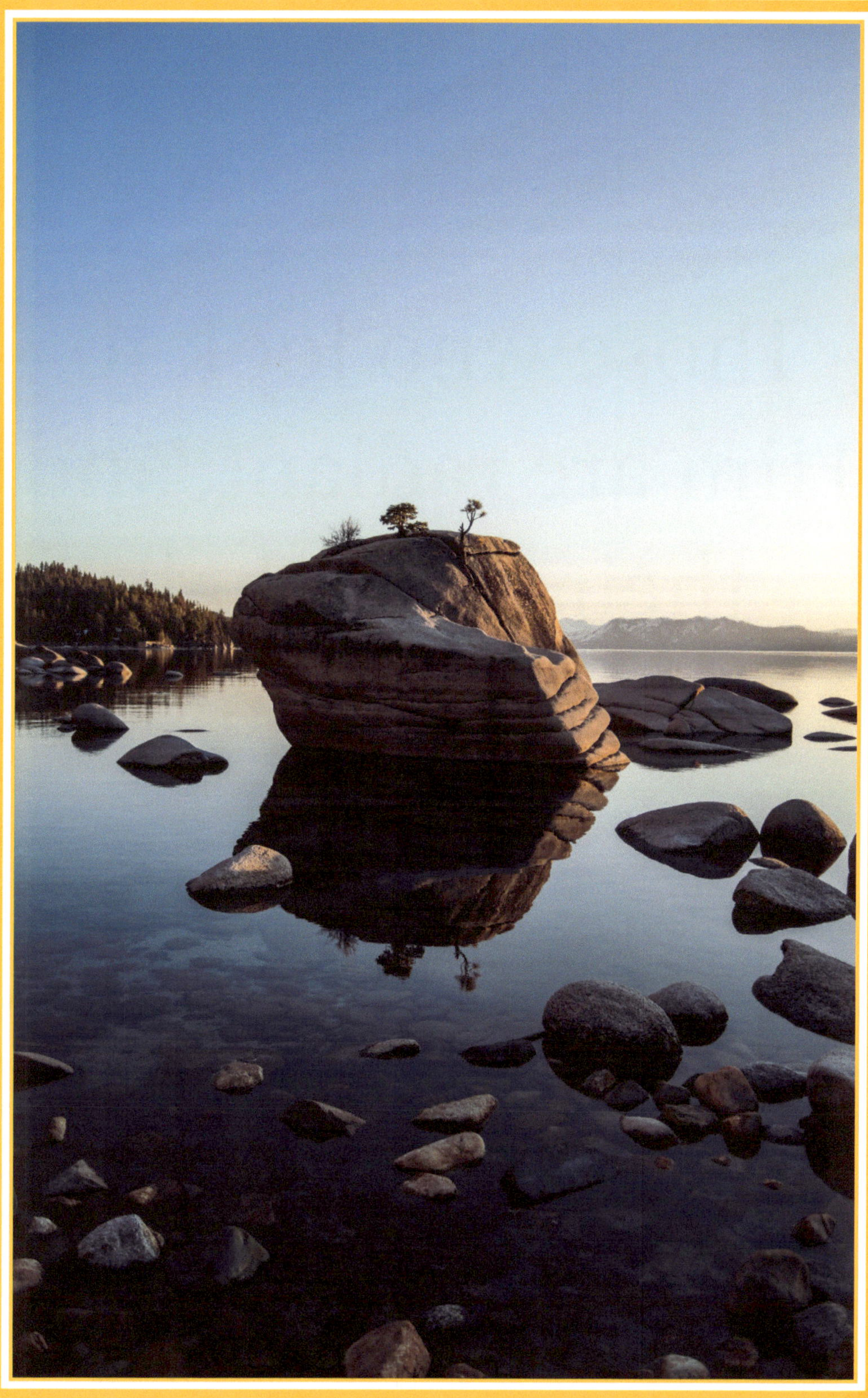

Those who look to Him are radiant, and their faces shall never be ashamed.

Psalm 34:5

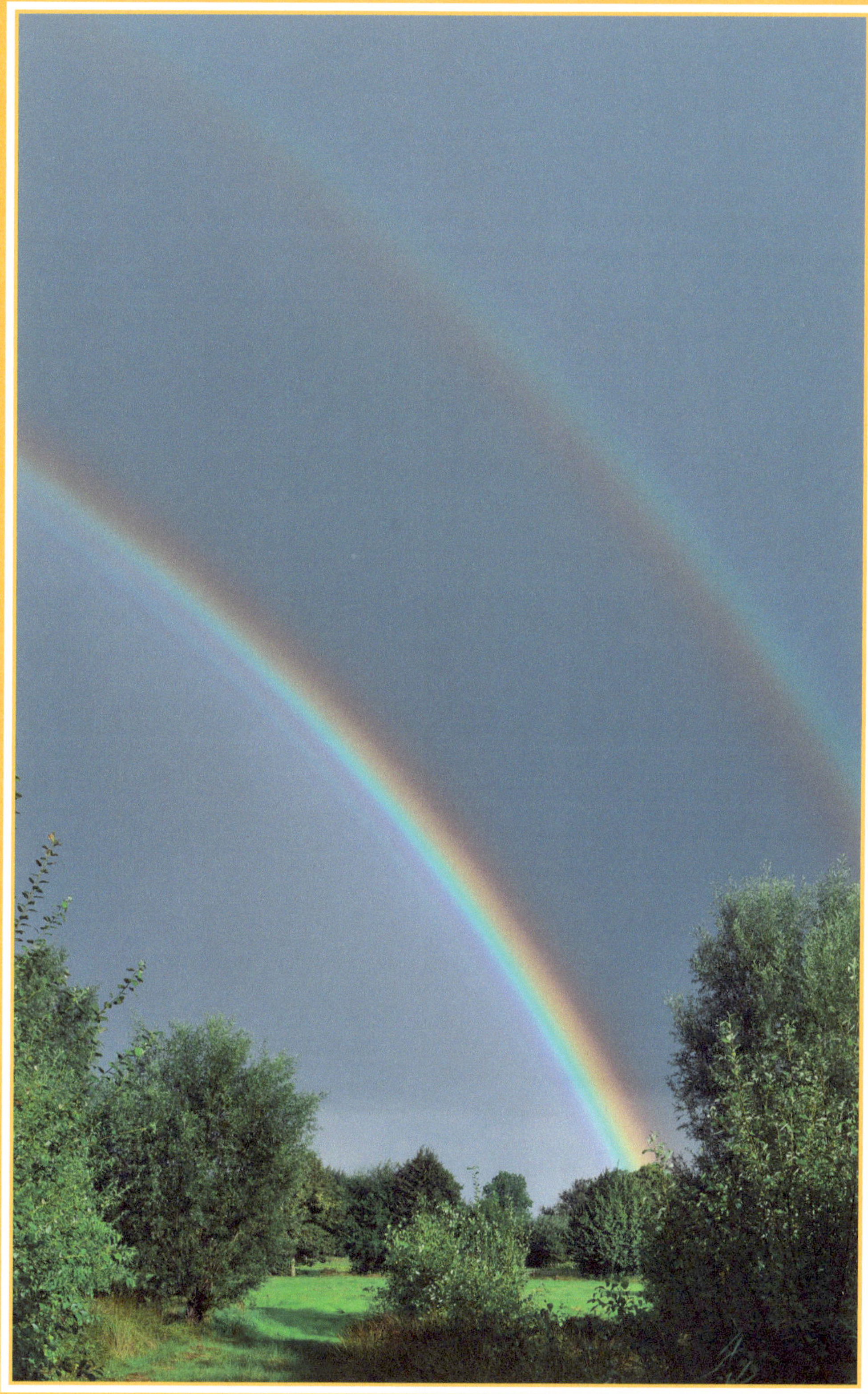

He will cover you
with his feathers.
He will shelter you
with his wings. His
faithful promises are
your armor and
protection.

Psalm 91:4

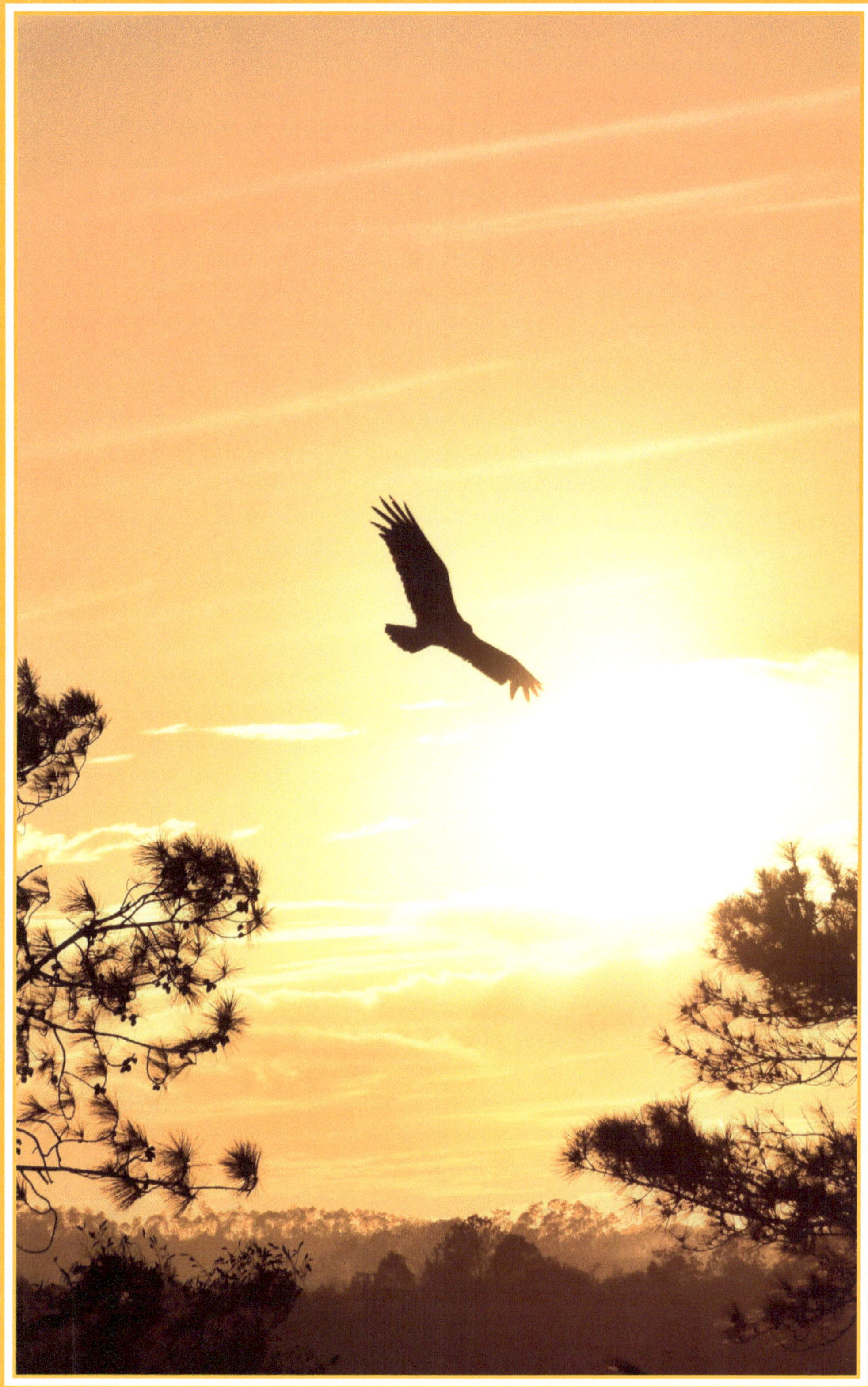

Delight yourself in
the LORD, and He
will give you the
desires of your heart.

Psalm 37:4

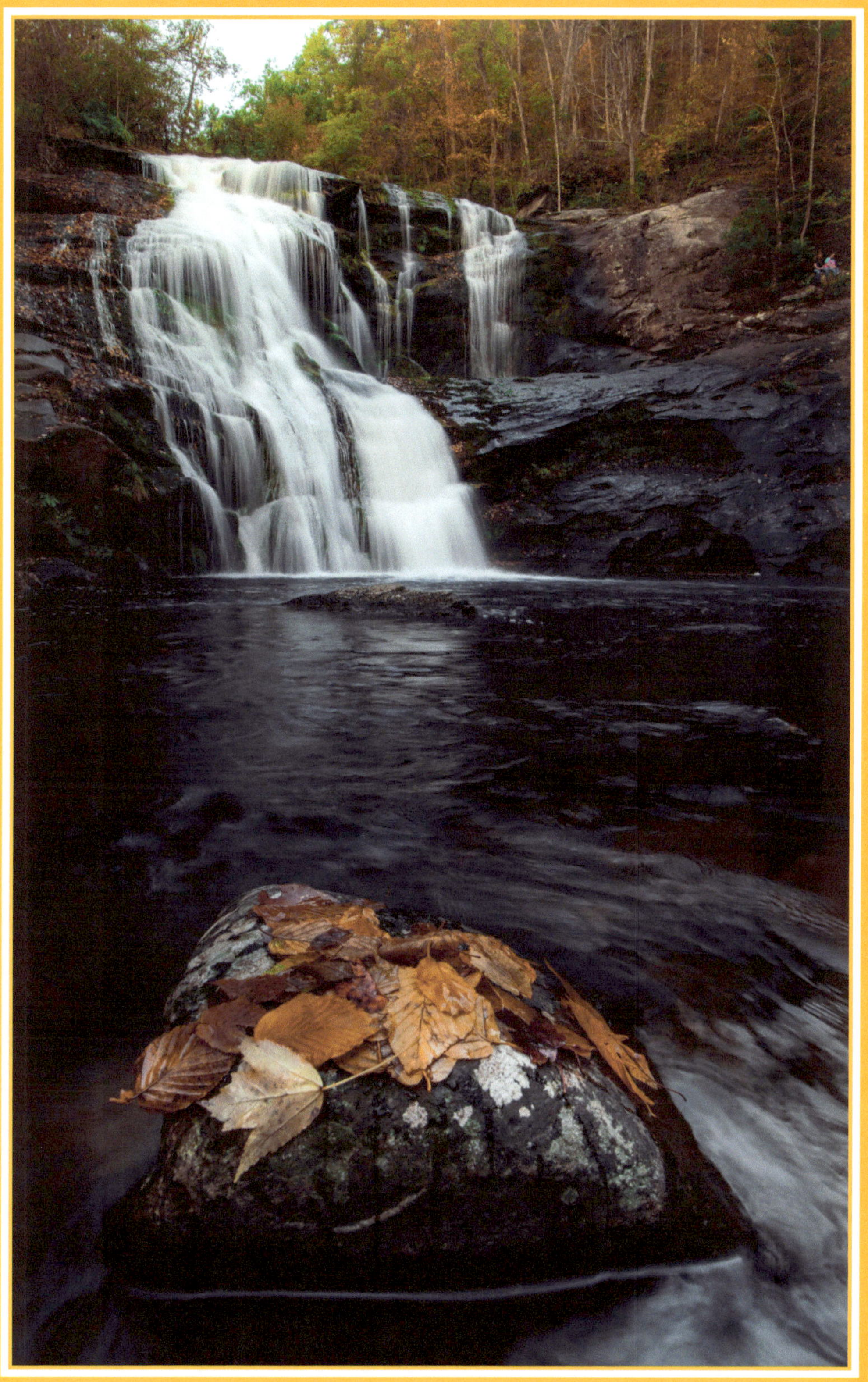

God is our refuge
and strength, an
ever-present help in
trouble.

Psalm 46:1

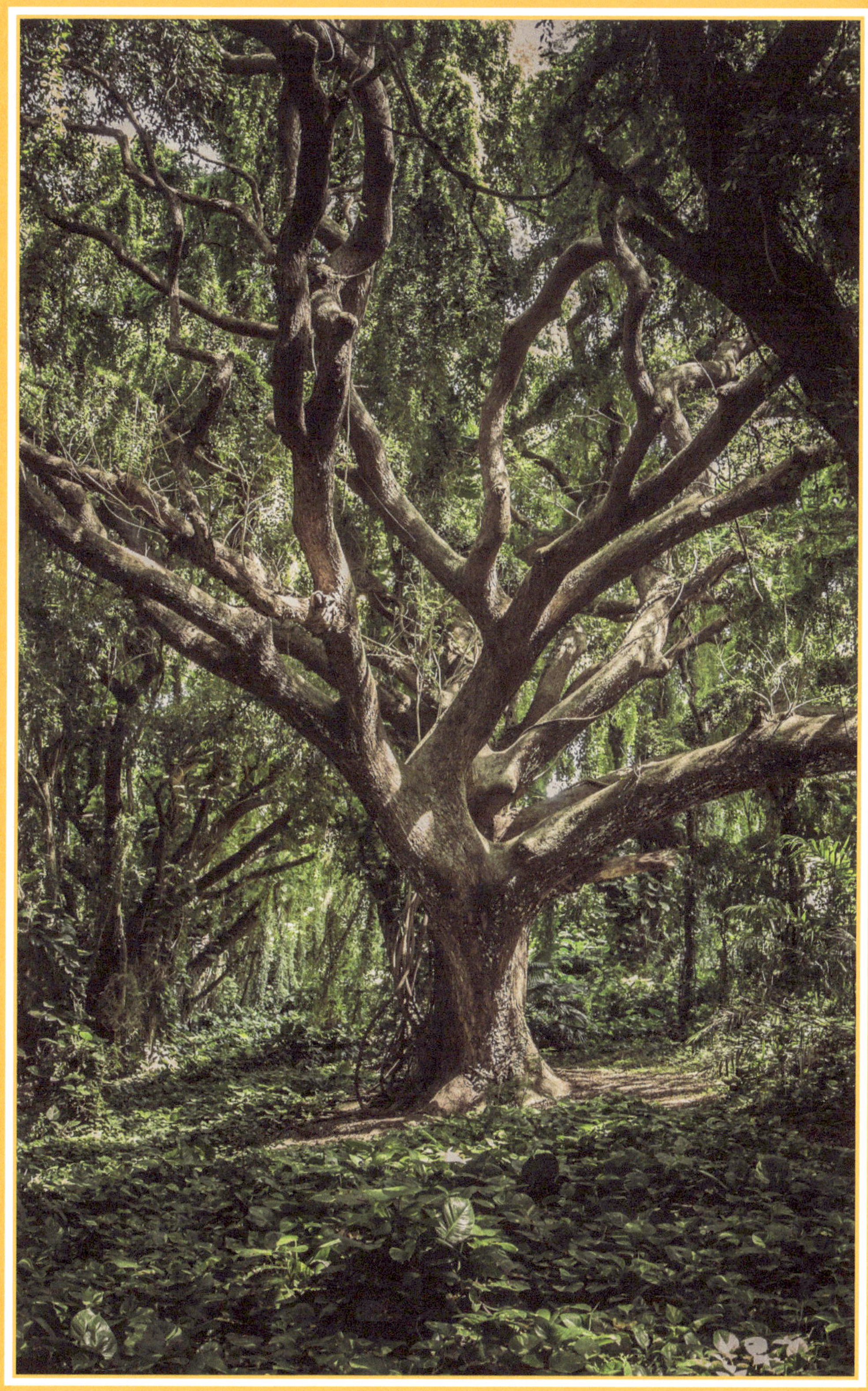

Your word is a lamp
for my feet, a light
on my path.

Psalm 119:105

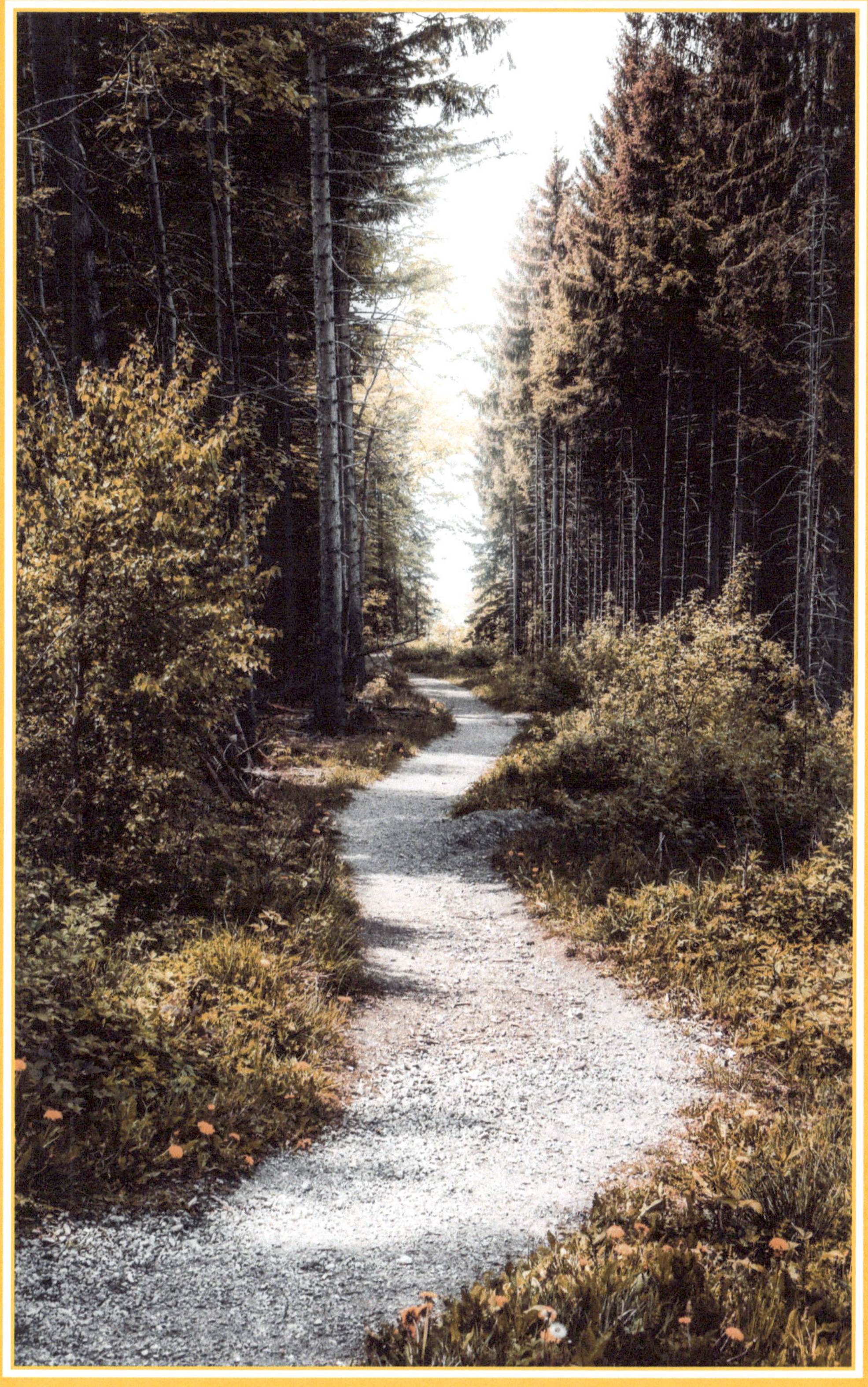

Be still and know
that I am God.

Psalm 46:10

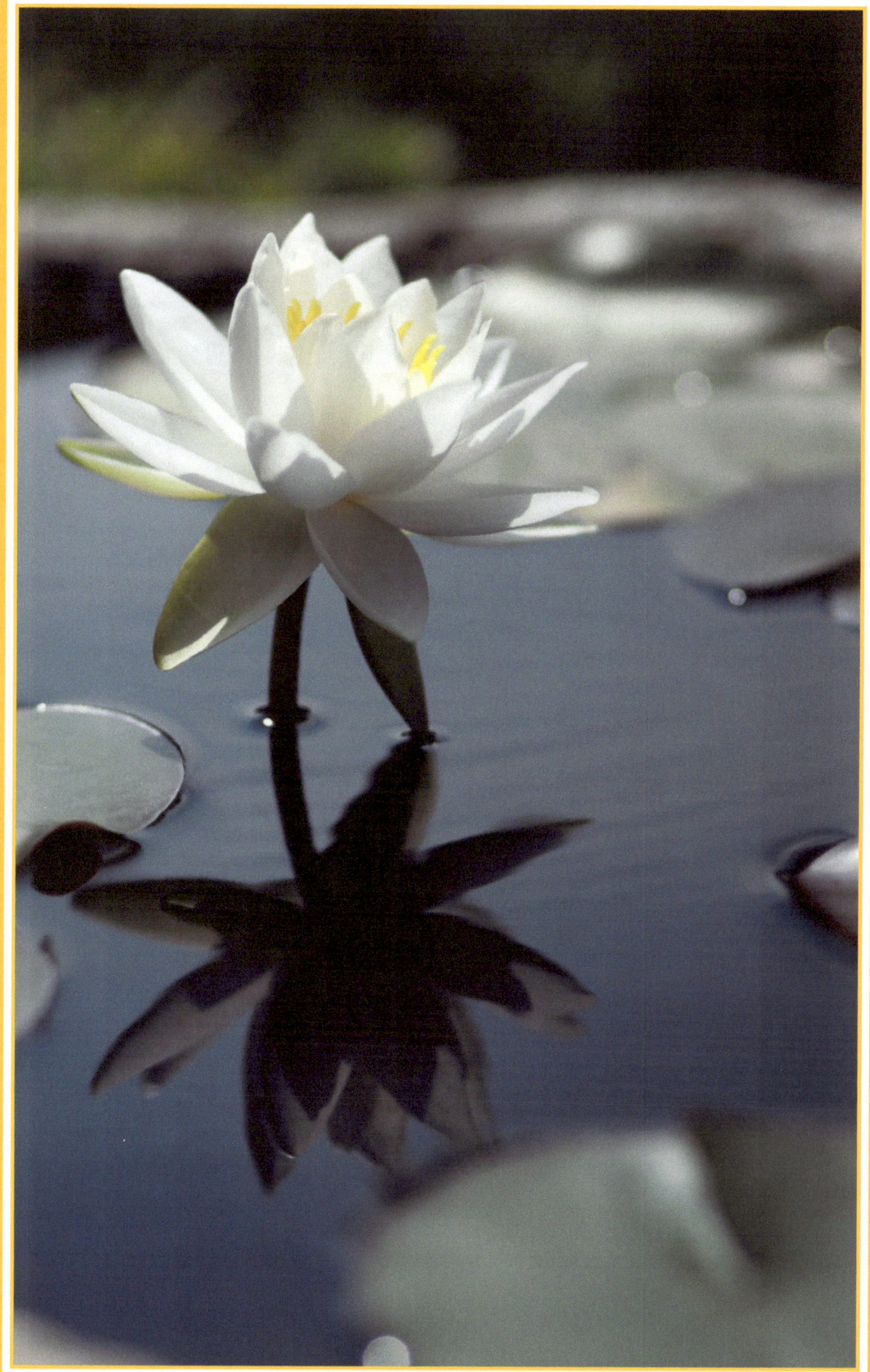

Cast your cares on
the LORD and he
will sustain you.

Psalm 55:22

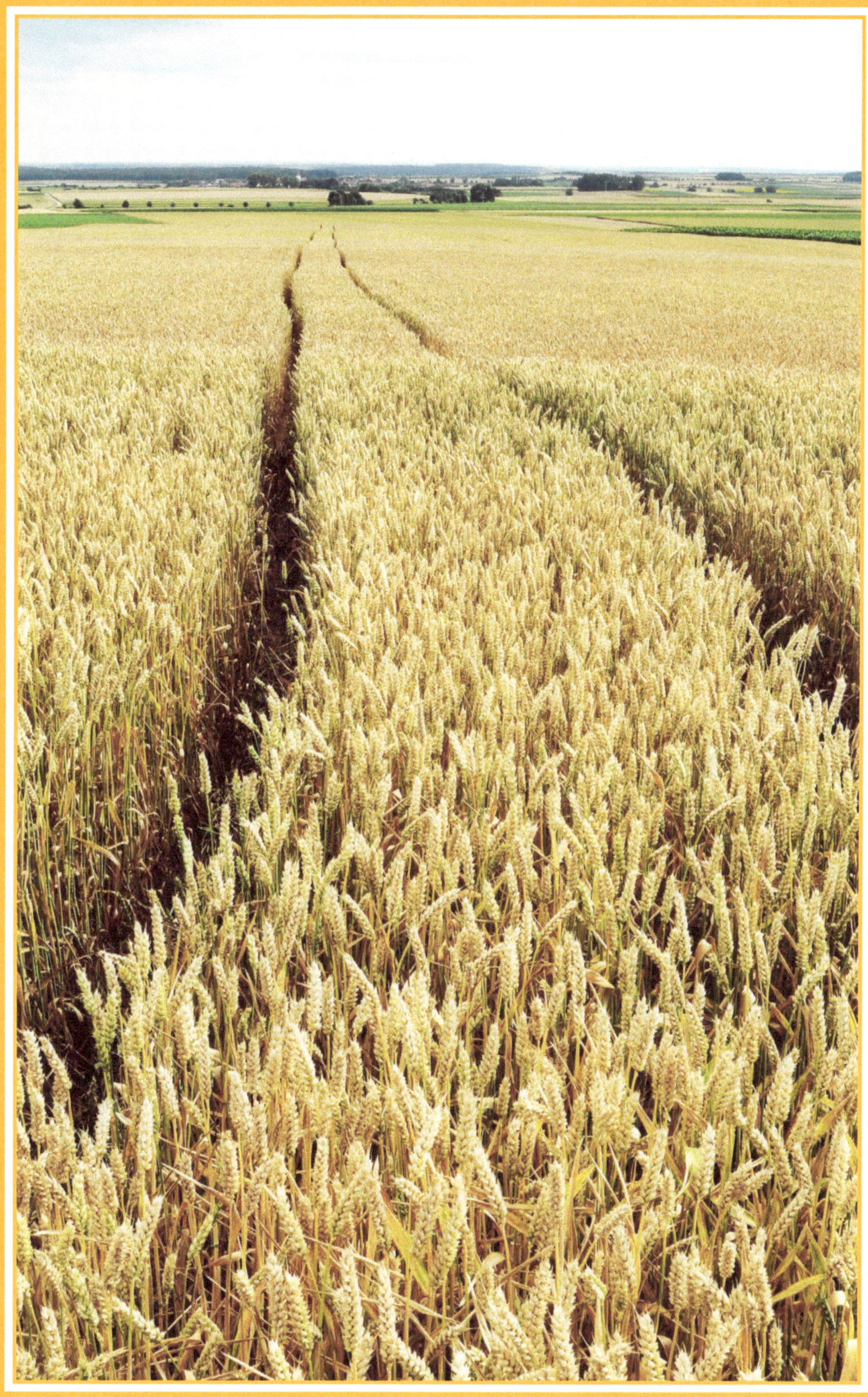

I keep my eyes
always on the
LORD. With him at
my right hand, I will
not be shaken.

Psalm 16:8

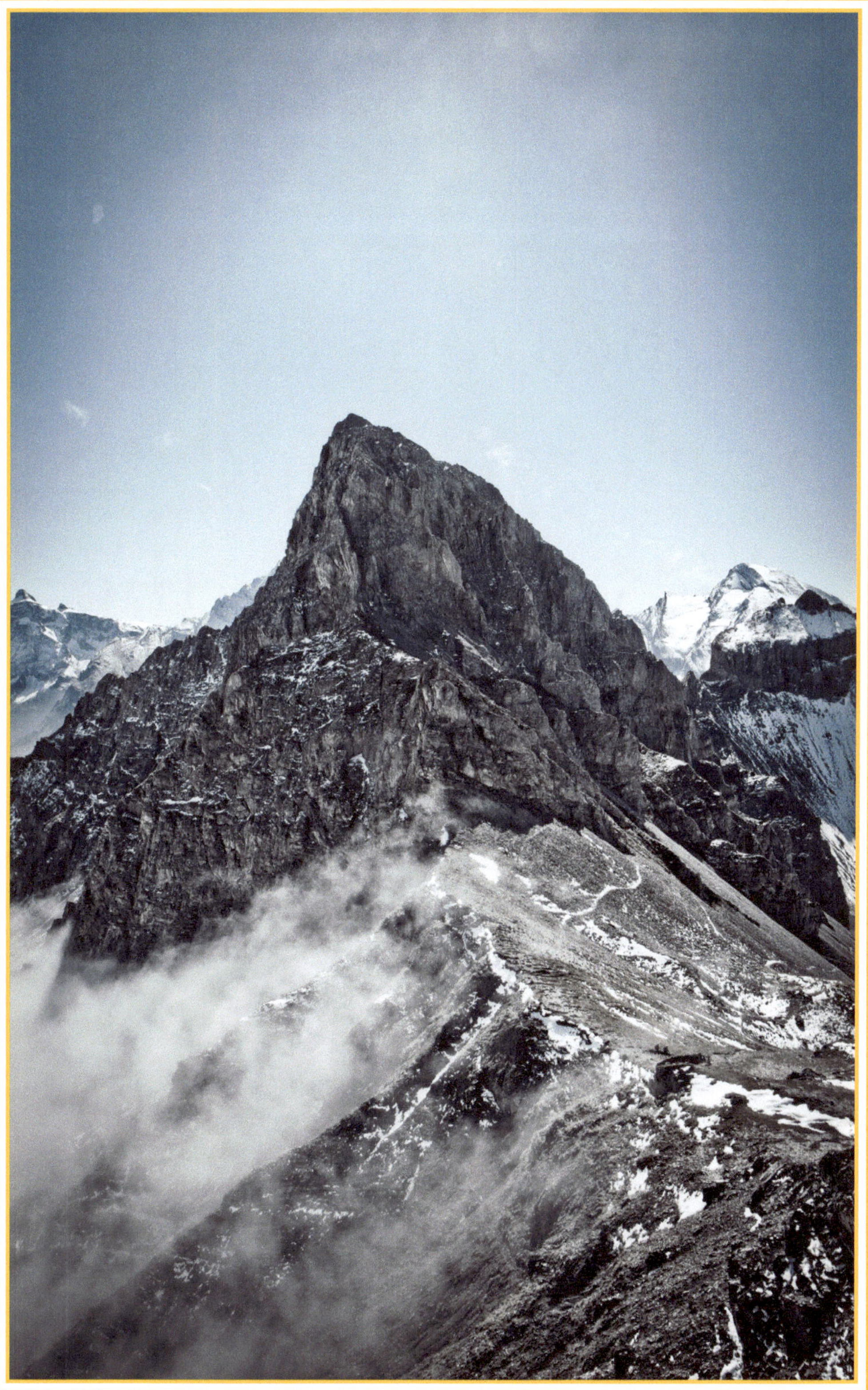

The heavens declare
the glory of God; the
skies proclaim the
work of his hands.

Psalm 19:1

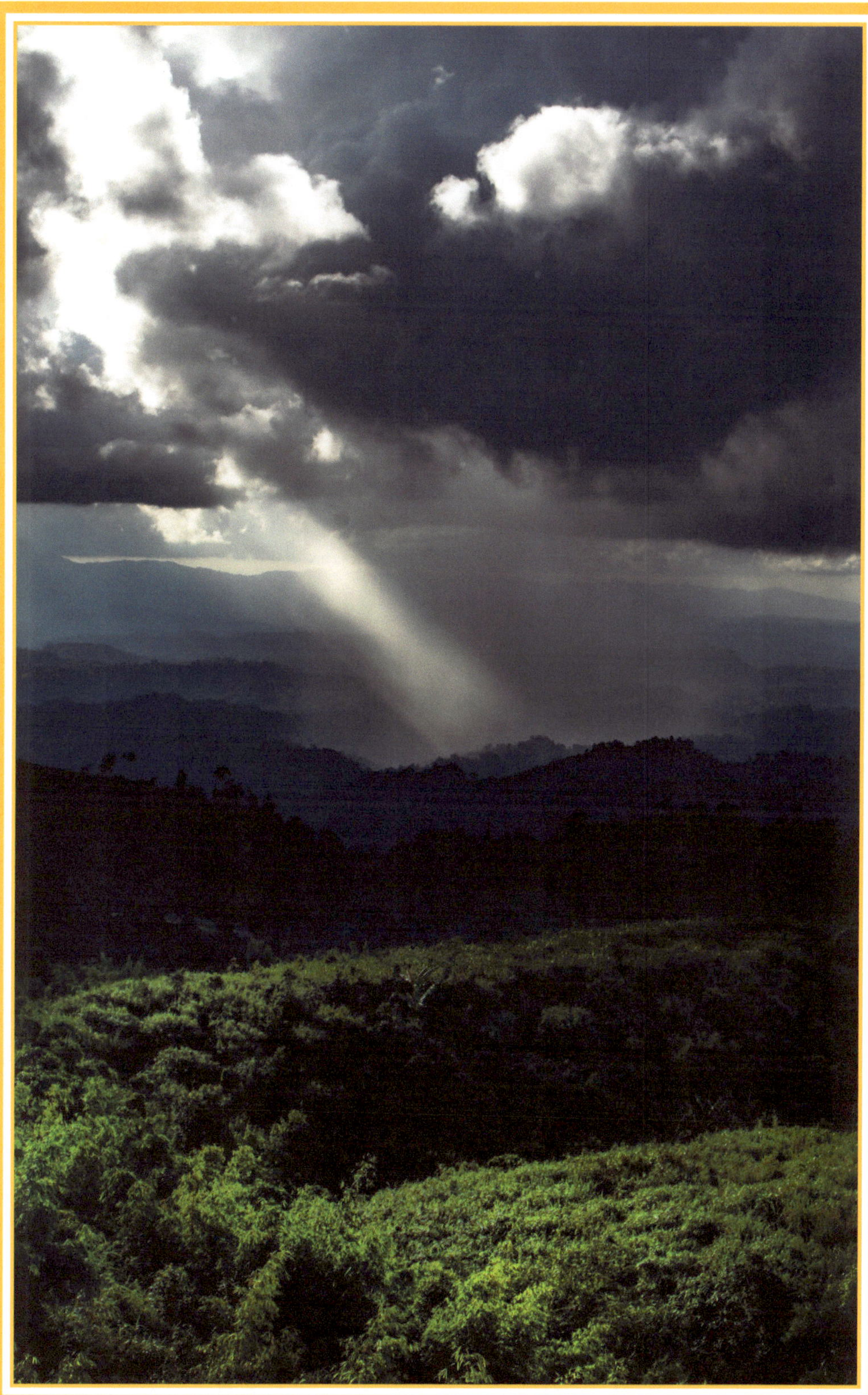

This is the day that the LORD has made; let us rejoice and be glad in it.

Psalm 118:24

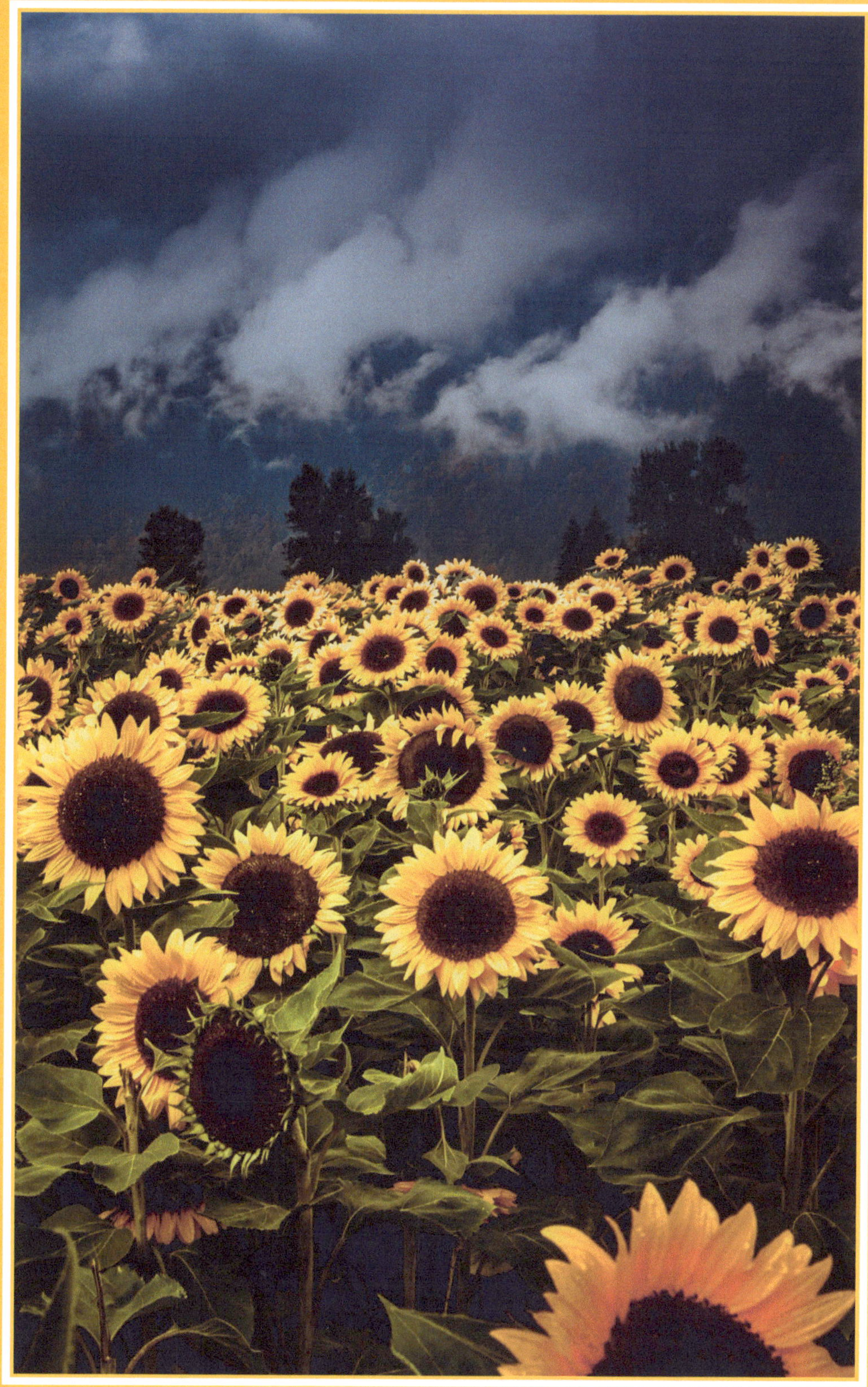

In peace I will lie down and sleep, for You alone, LORD, make me dwell in safety.

Psalm 4:8

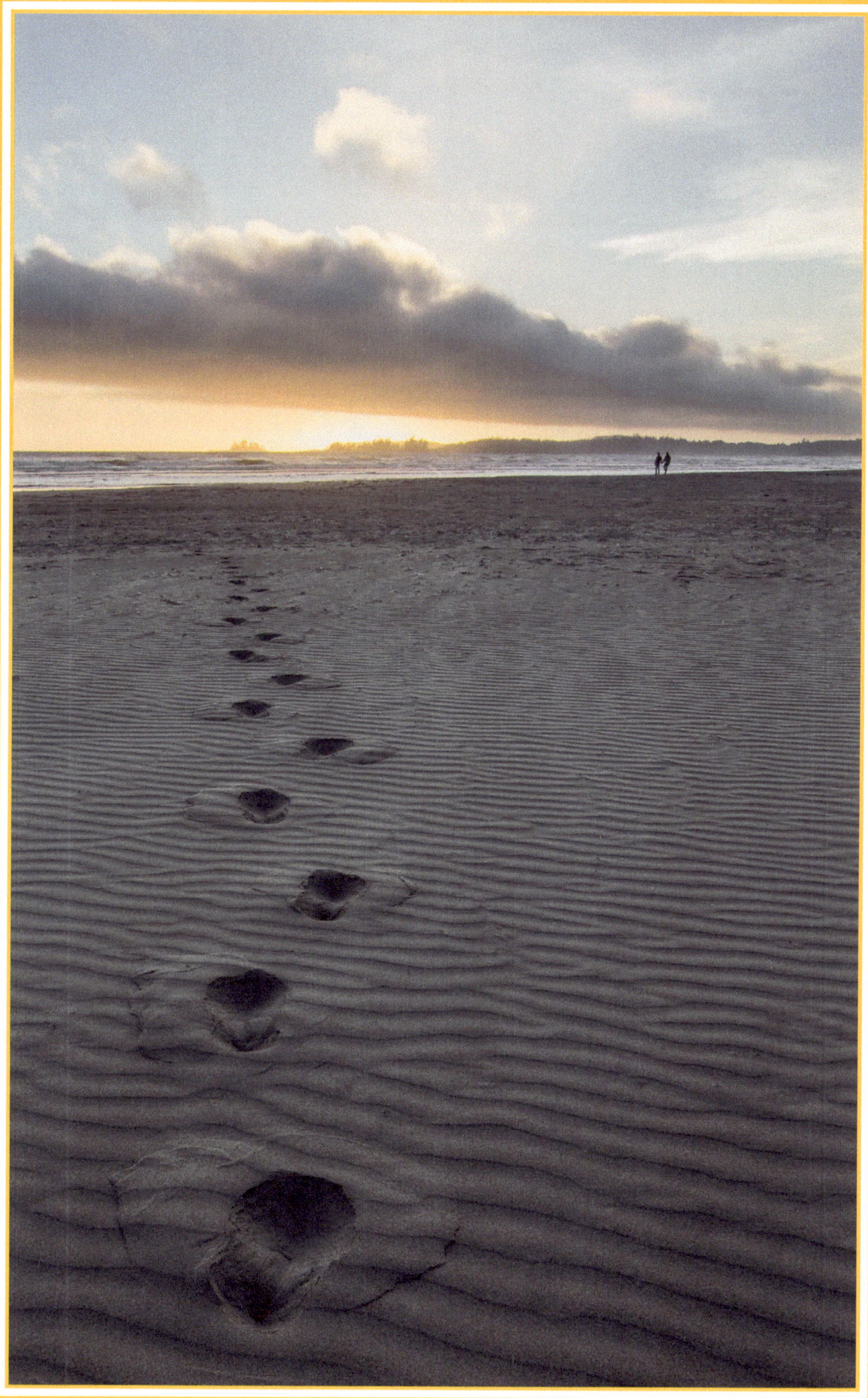

You make known to me the path of life; You will fill me with joy in Your presence, with eternal pleasures at Your right hand.

Psalm 16:11

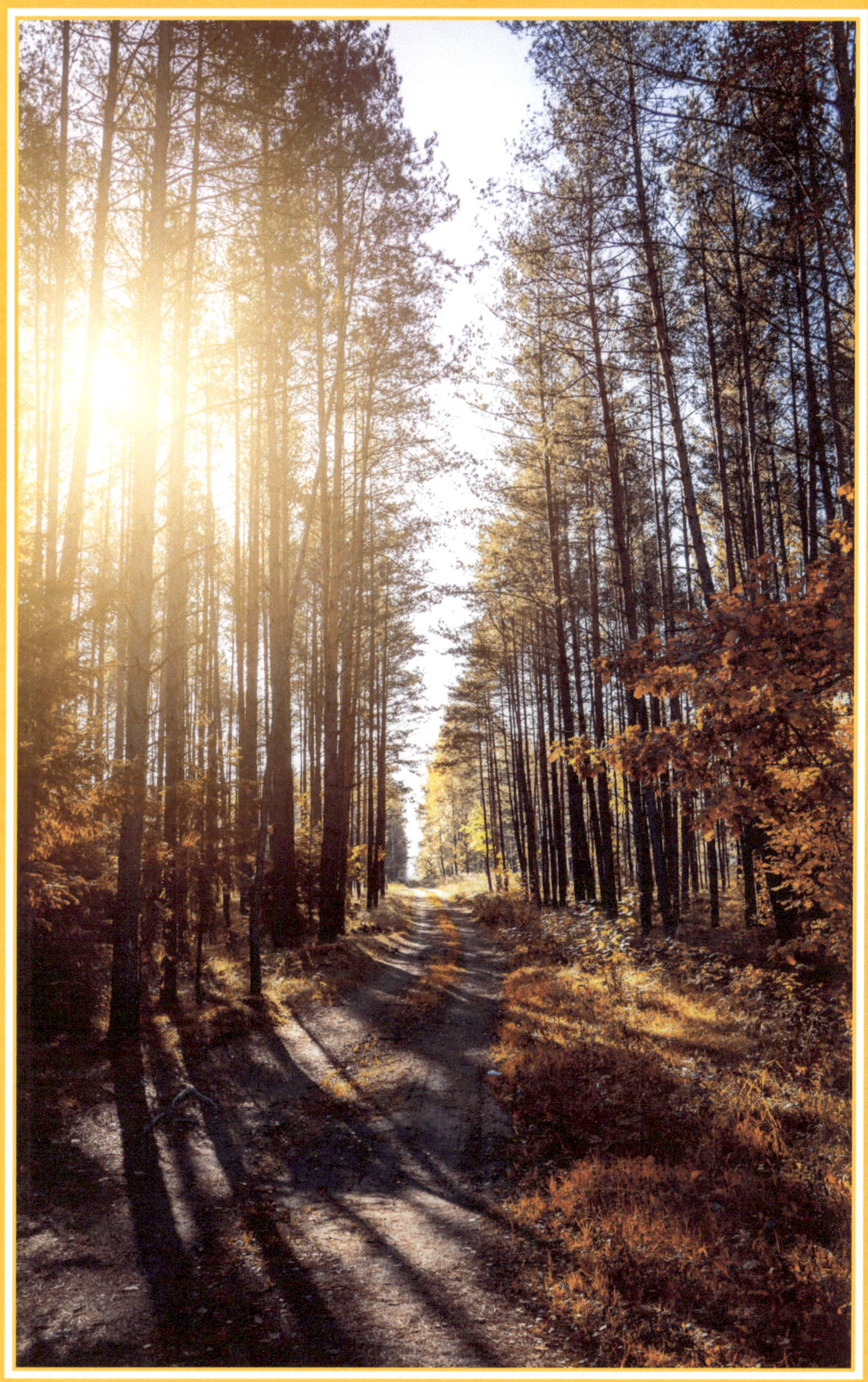

LORD my God, I called to You for help, and You healed me.

Psalm 30:2

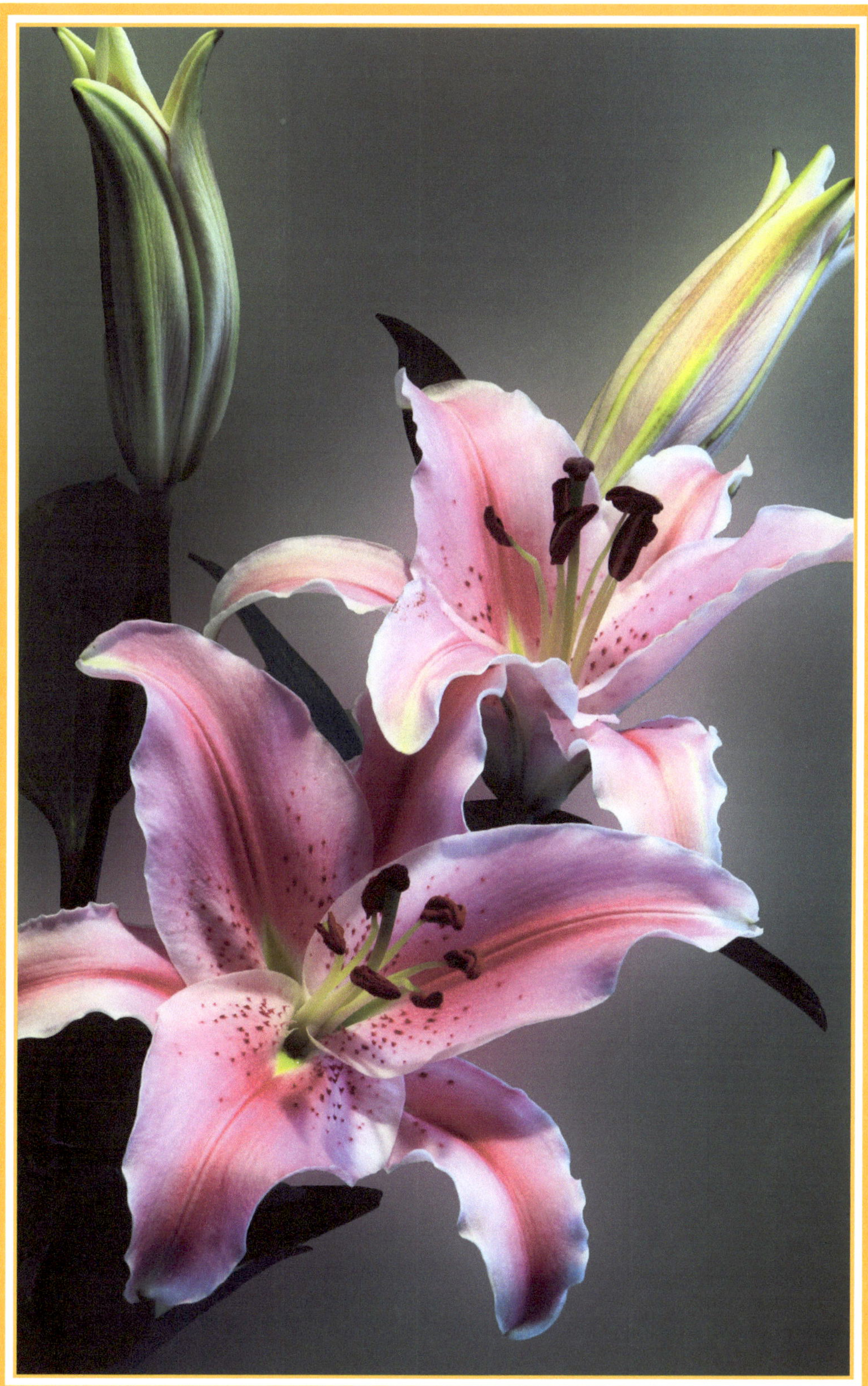

But I trust in Your unfailing love; my heart rejoices in Your salvation.

Psalm 13:5

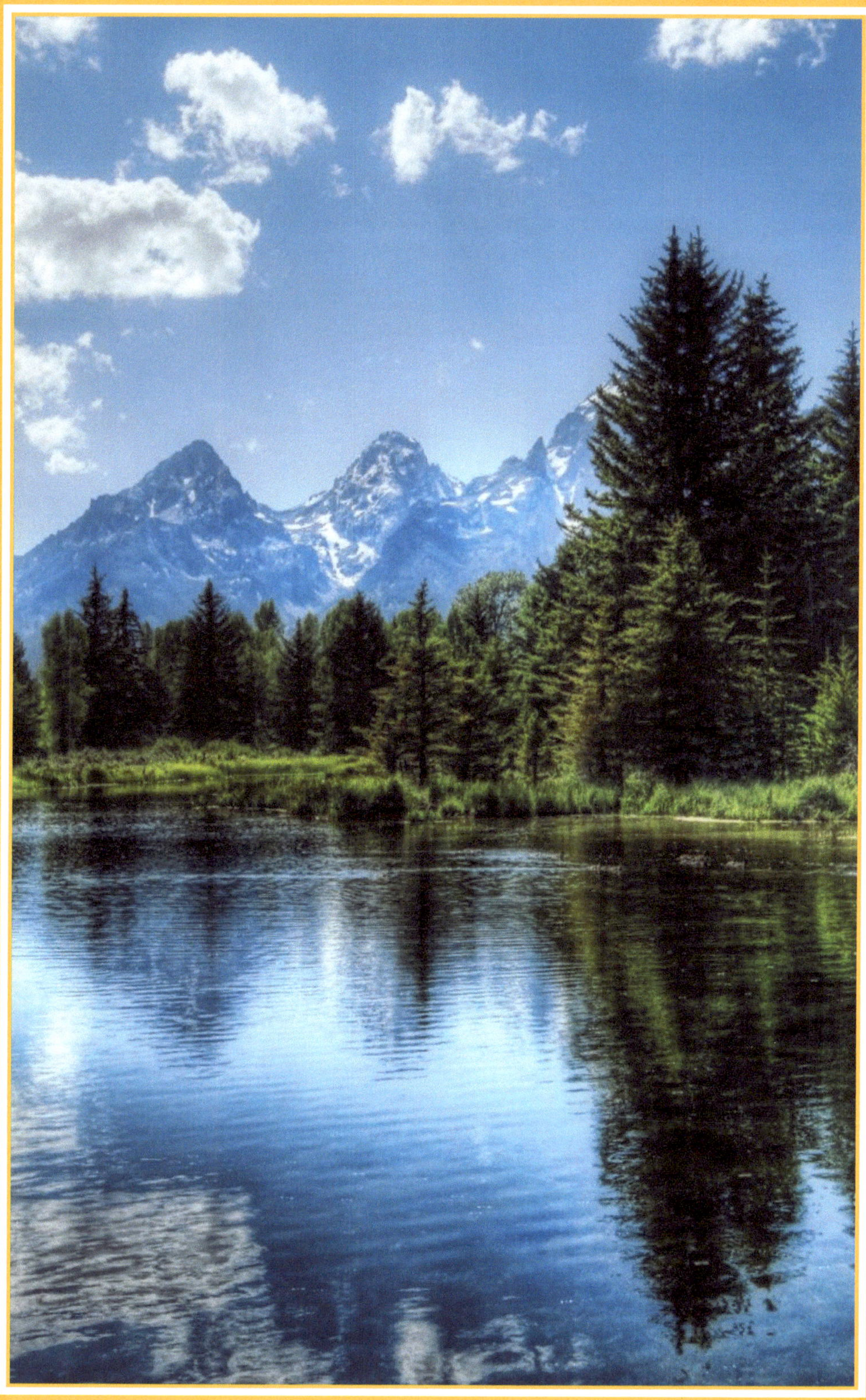

In you, LORD my God, I put my trust.

Psalm 25:1

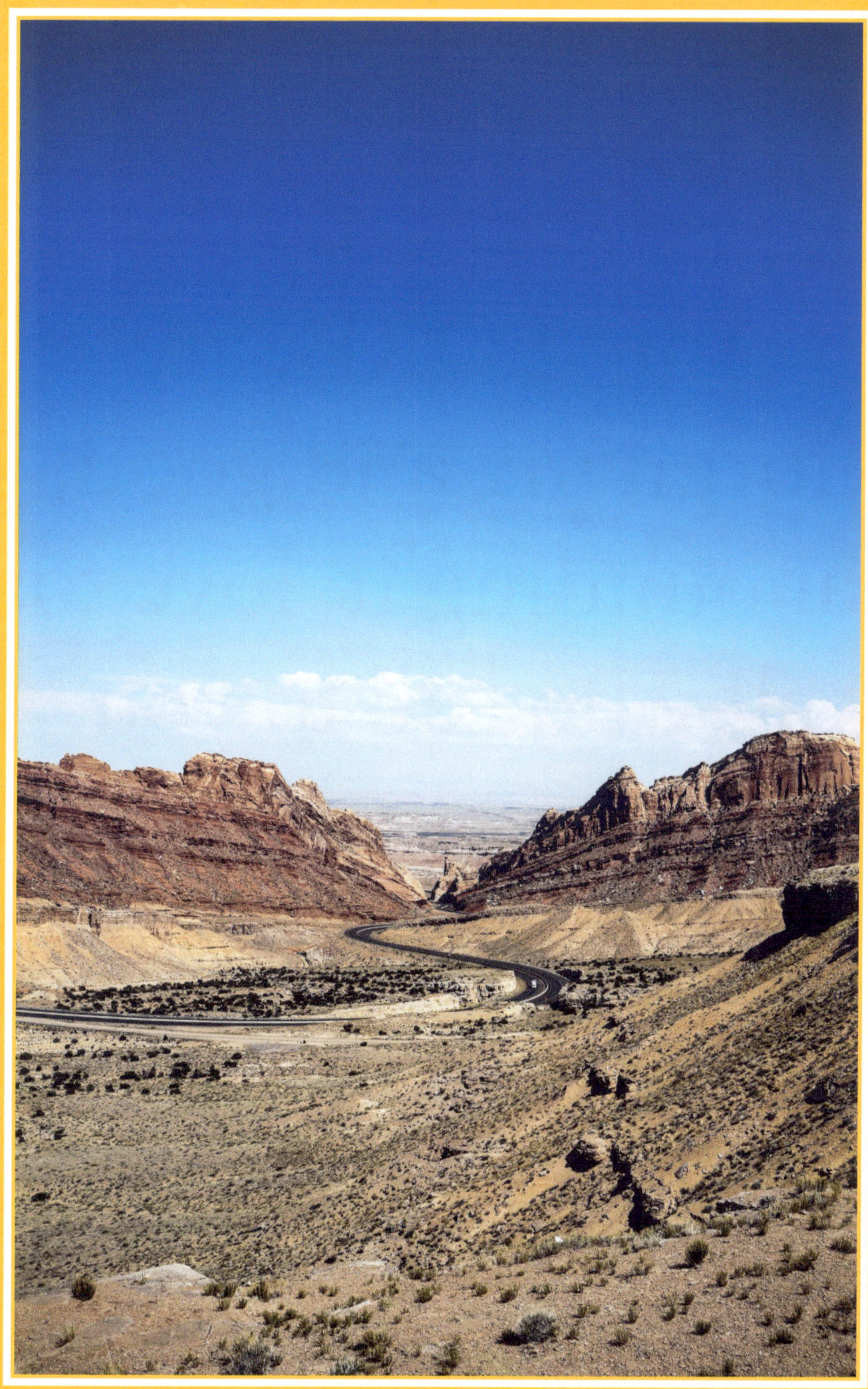

You, LORD, are forgiving and good, abounding in love to all who call to you.

Psalm 86:5

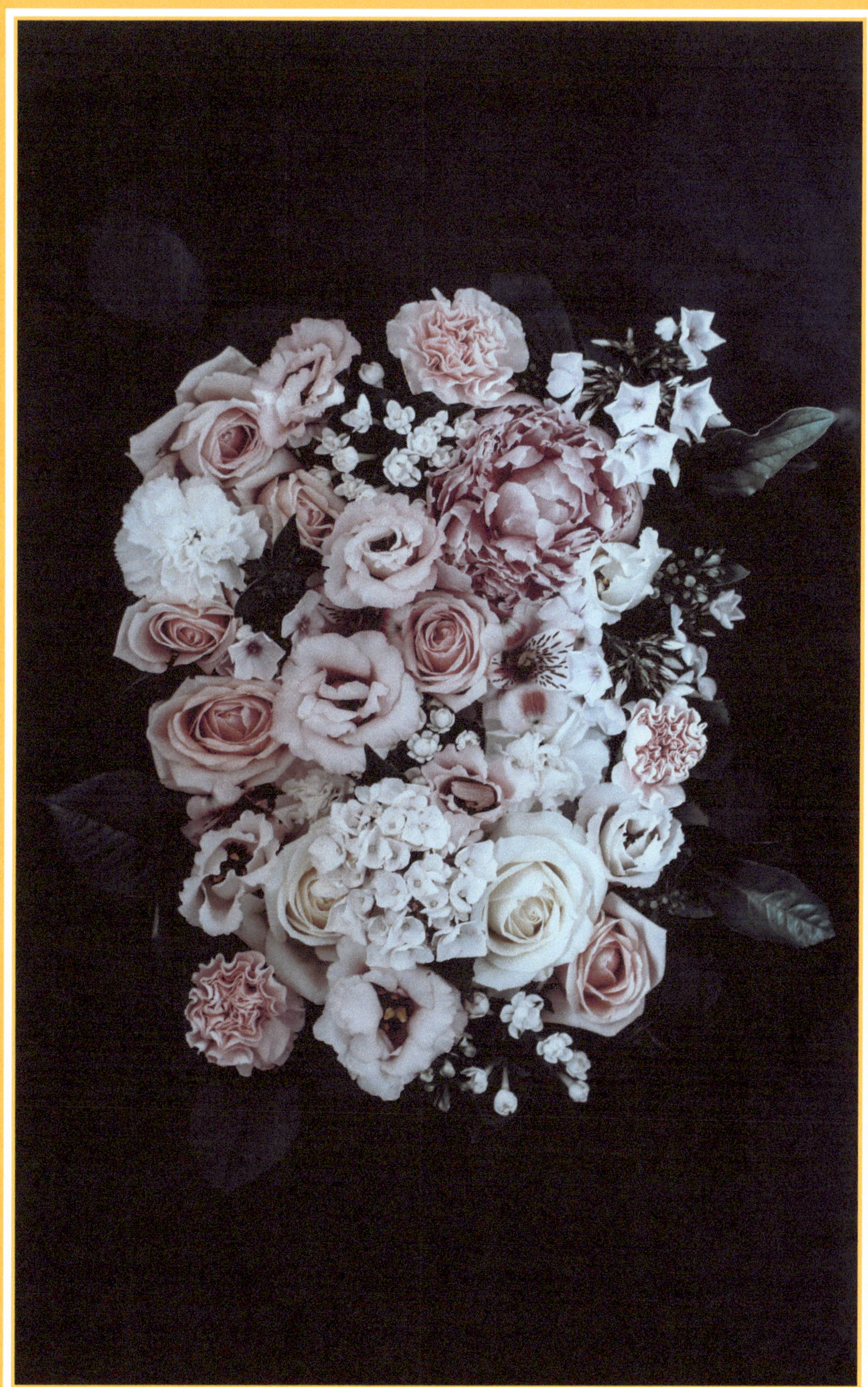

The LORD has done
great things for
us, and we are filled
with joy.

Psalm 126:3

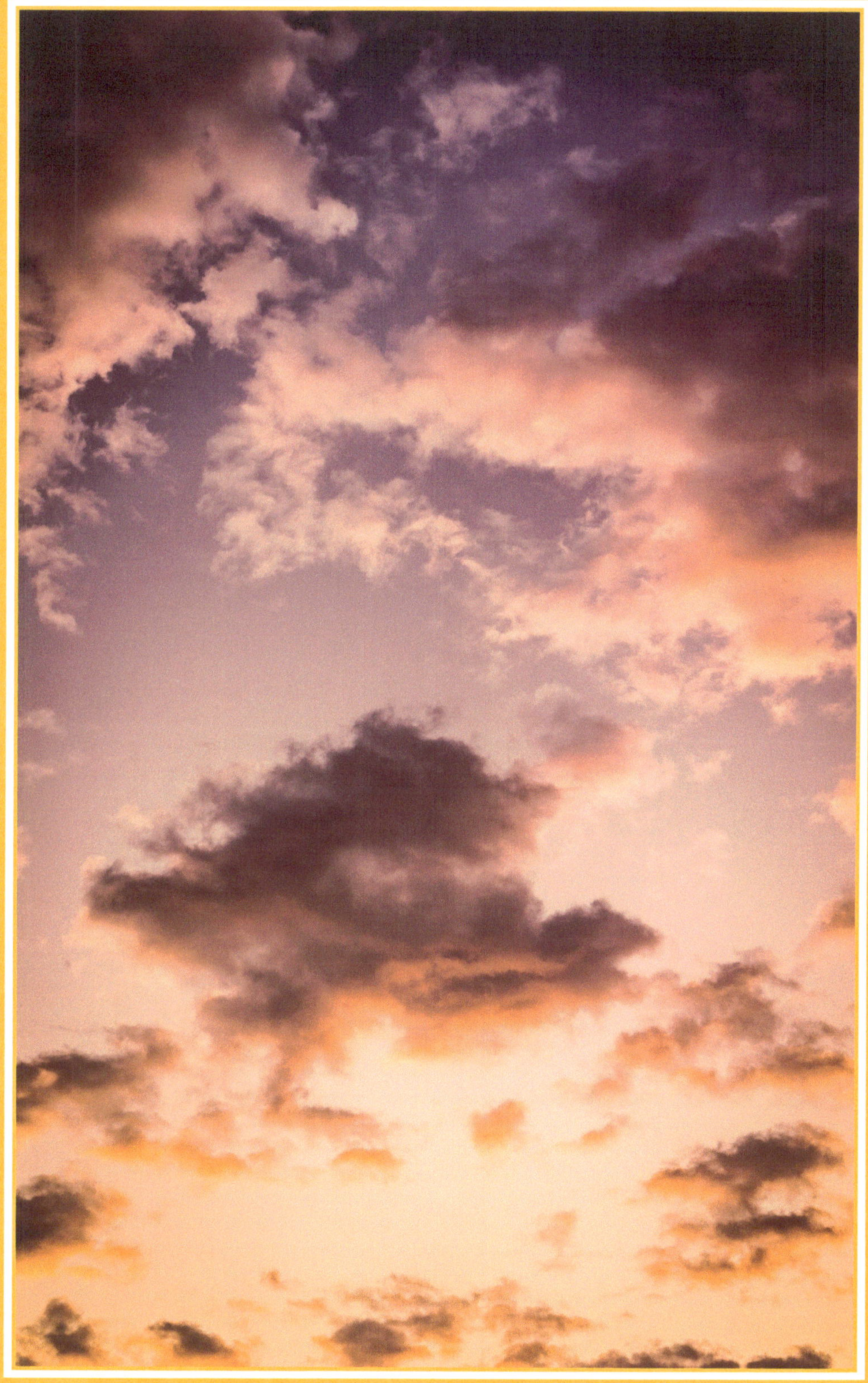

I will give thanks to
You, LORD, with all
my heart; I will
tell of all Your
wonderful deeds.

Psalm 9:1

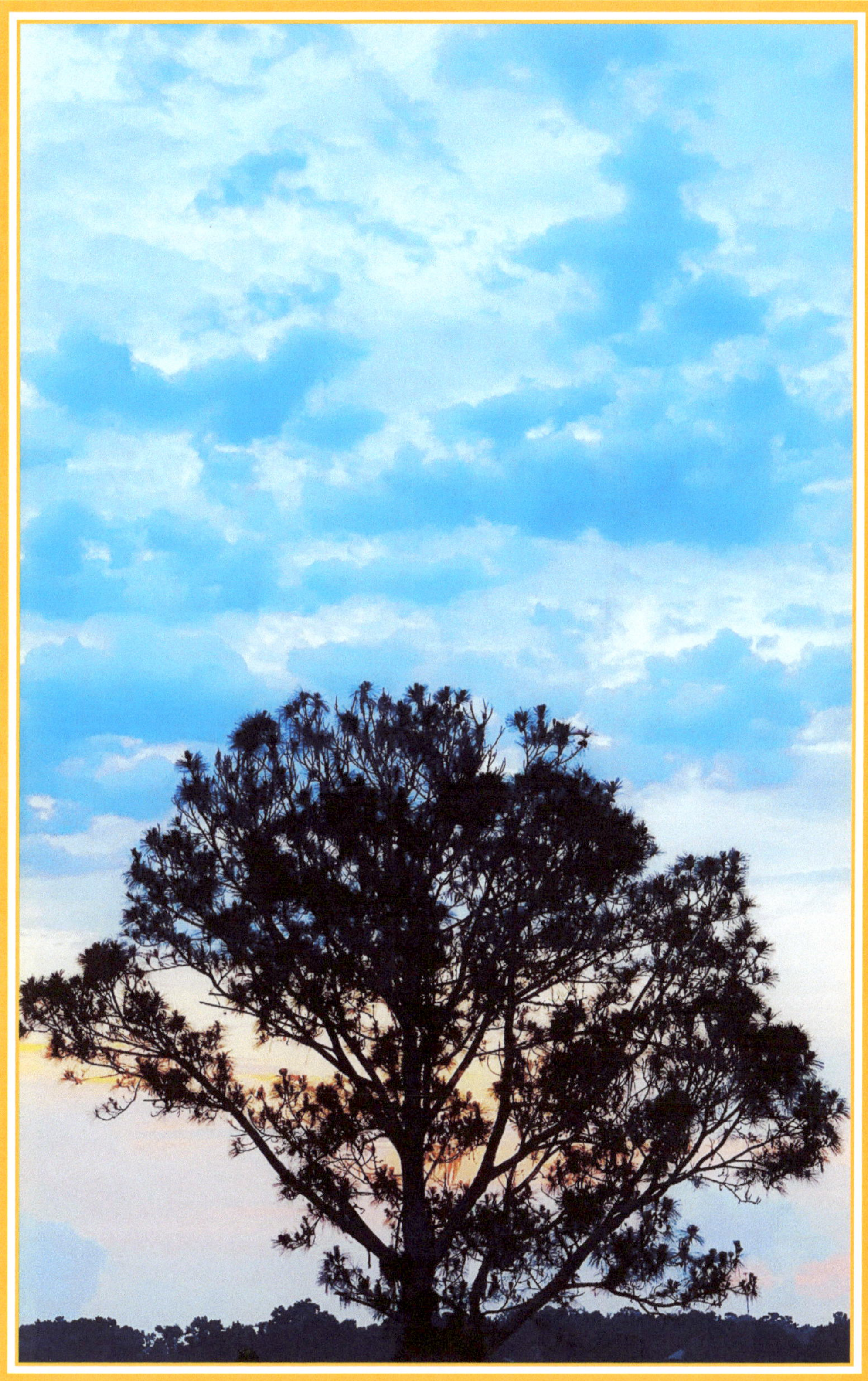

Keep me safe, my
God, for in you I
take refuge.

Psalm 16:1

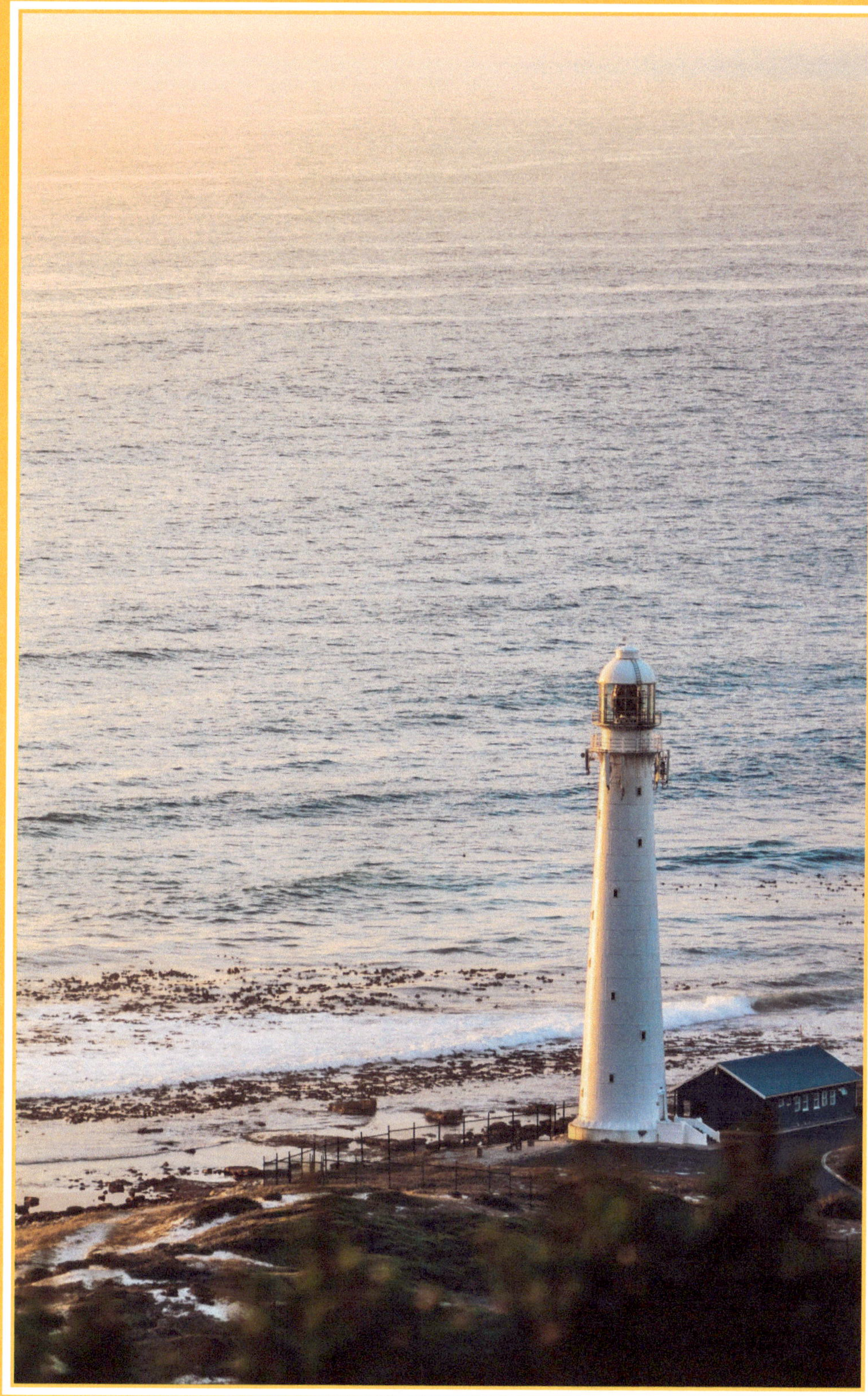

The earth is
the LORD's, and
everything in it, the
world, and all who
live in it.

Psalm 24:1

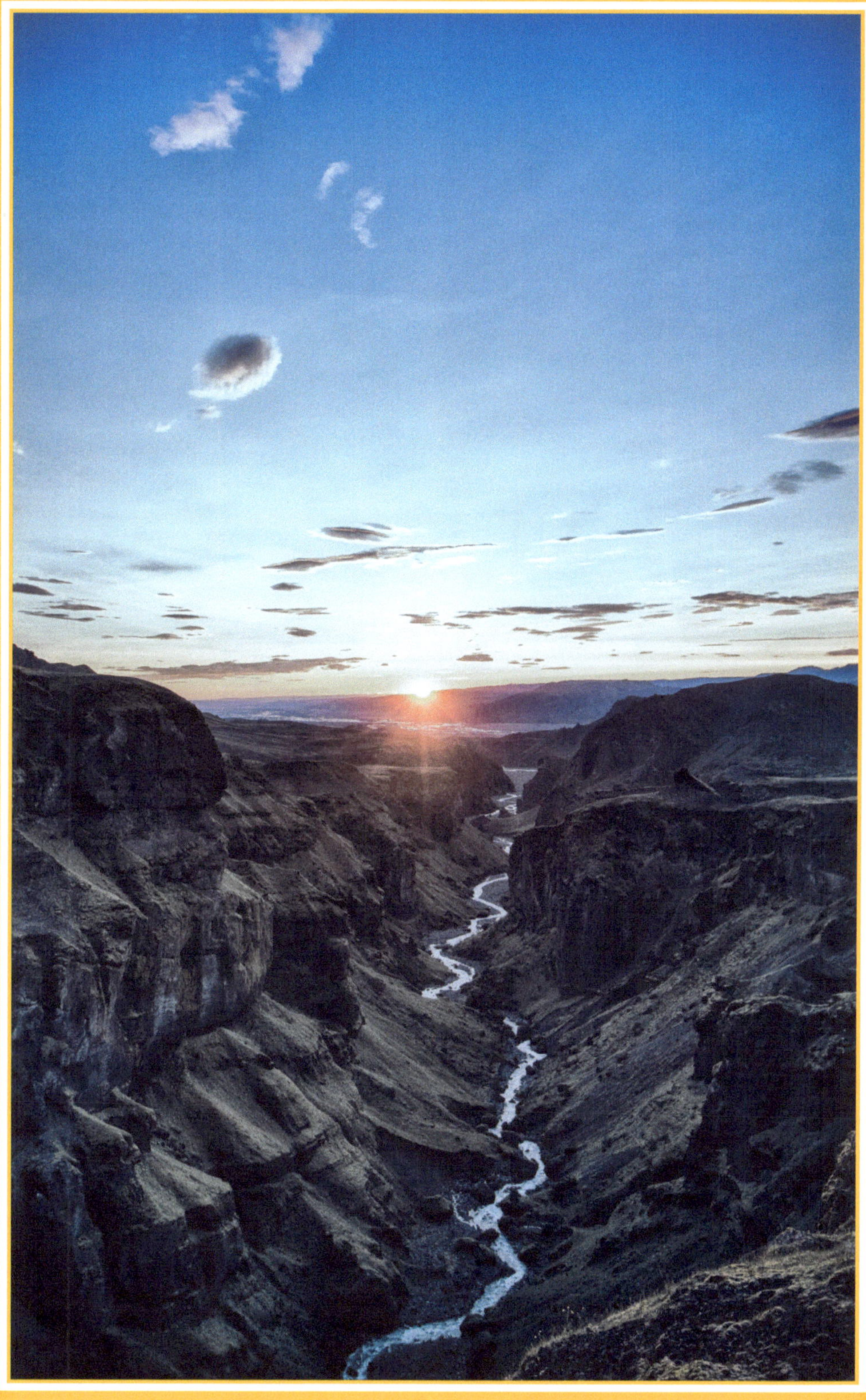

Shout for joy to God, all the earth!

Psalms 66:1

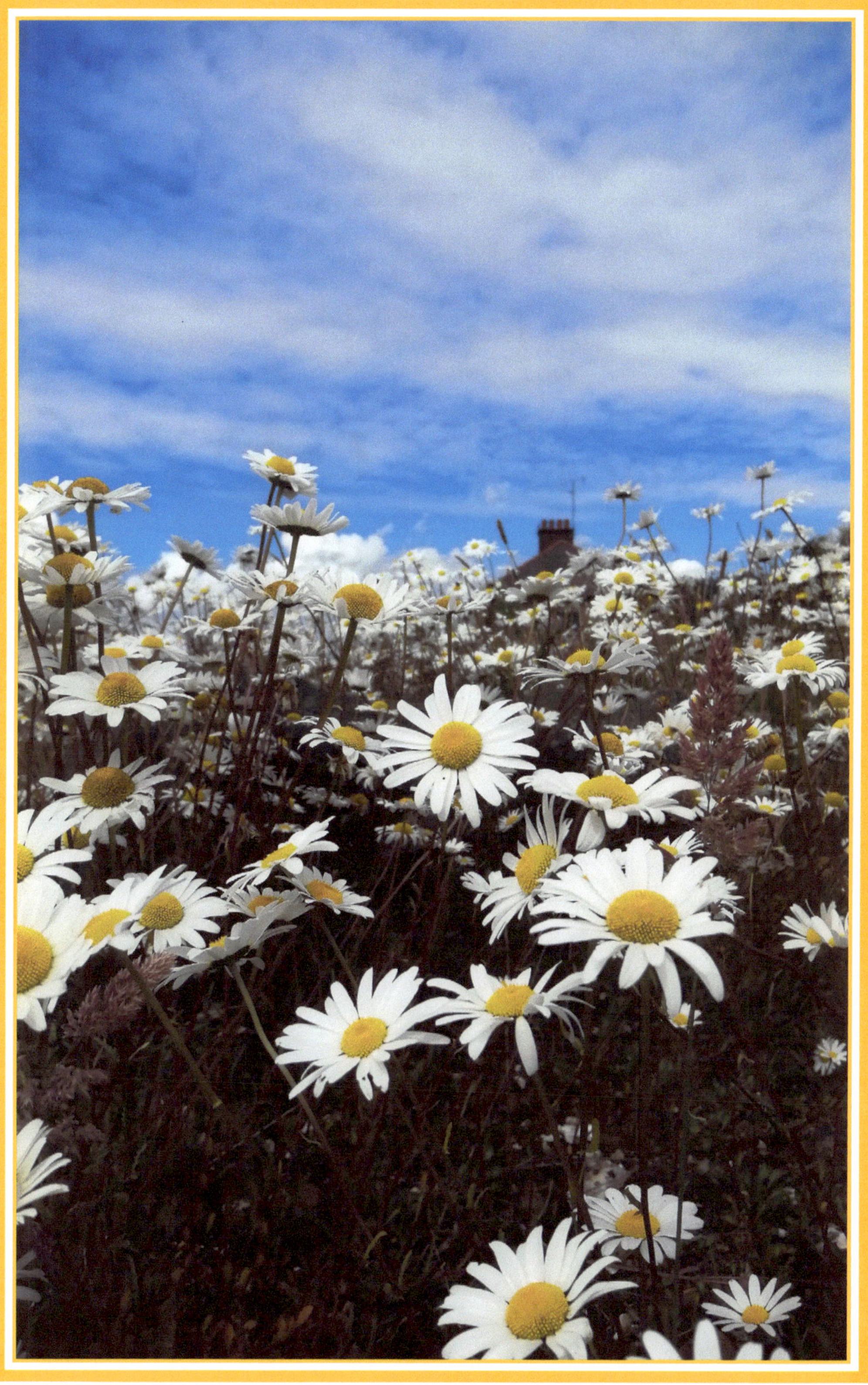

I will
sing the LORD's
praise, for he has
been good to me.

Psalm 13:6

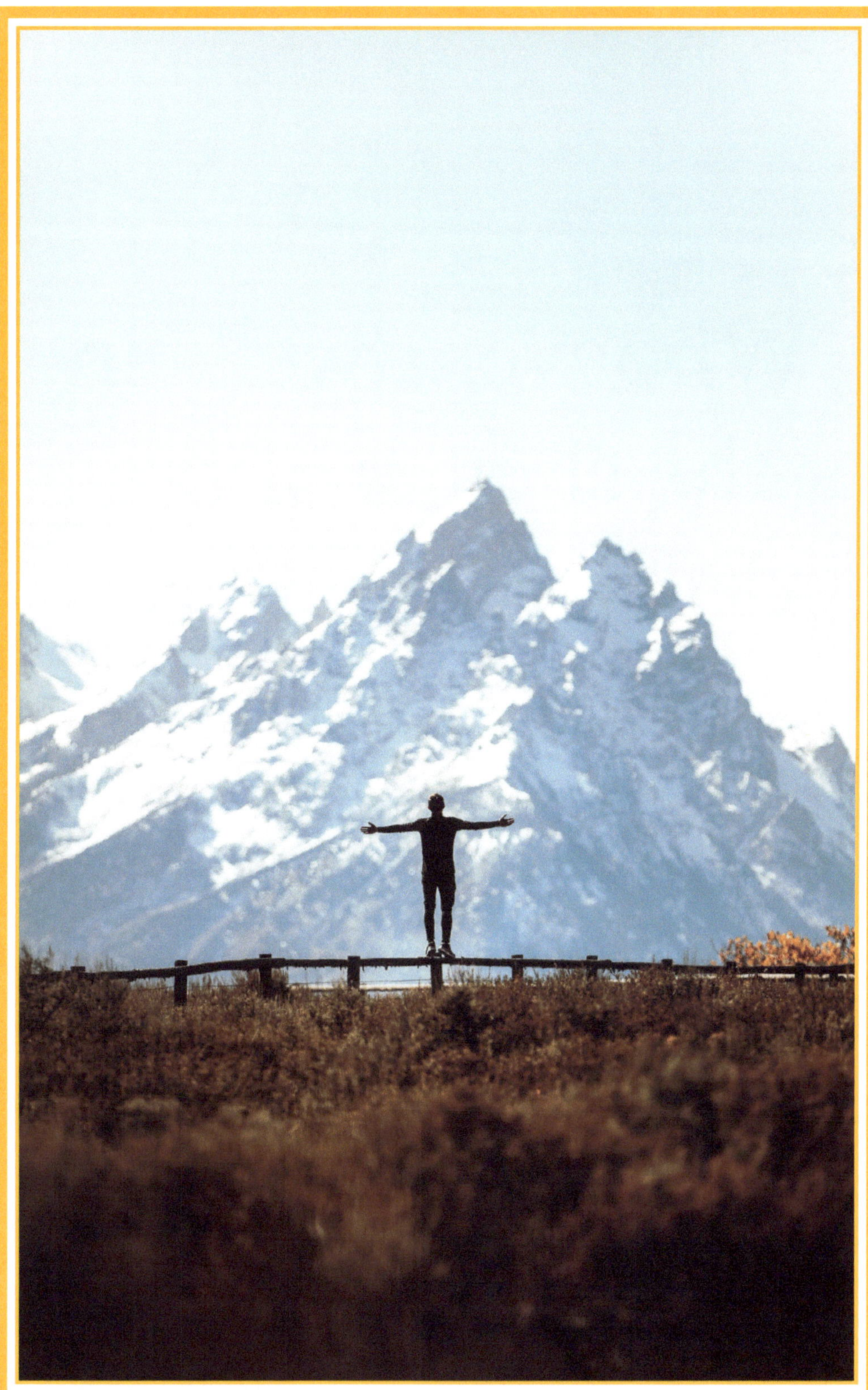

Whoever dwells in
the shelter of the
Most High will rest
in the shadow of the
Almighty.

Psalm 91:1

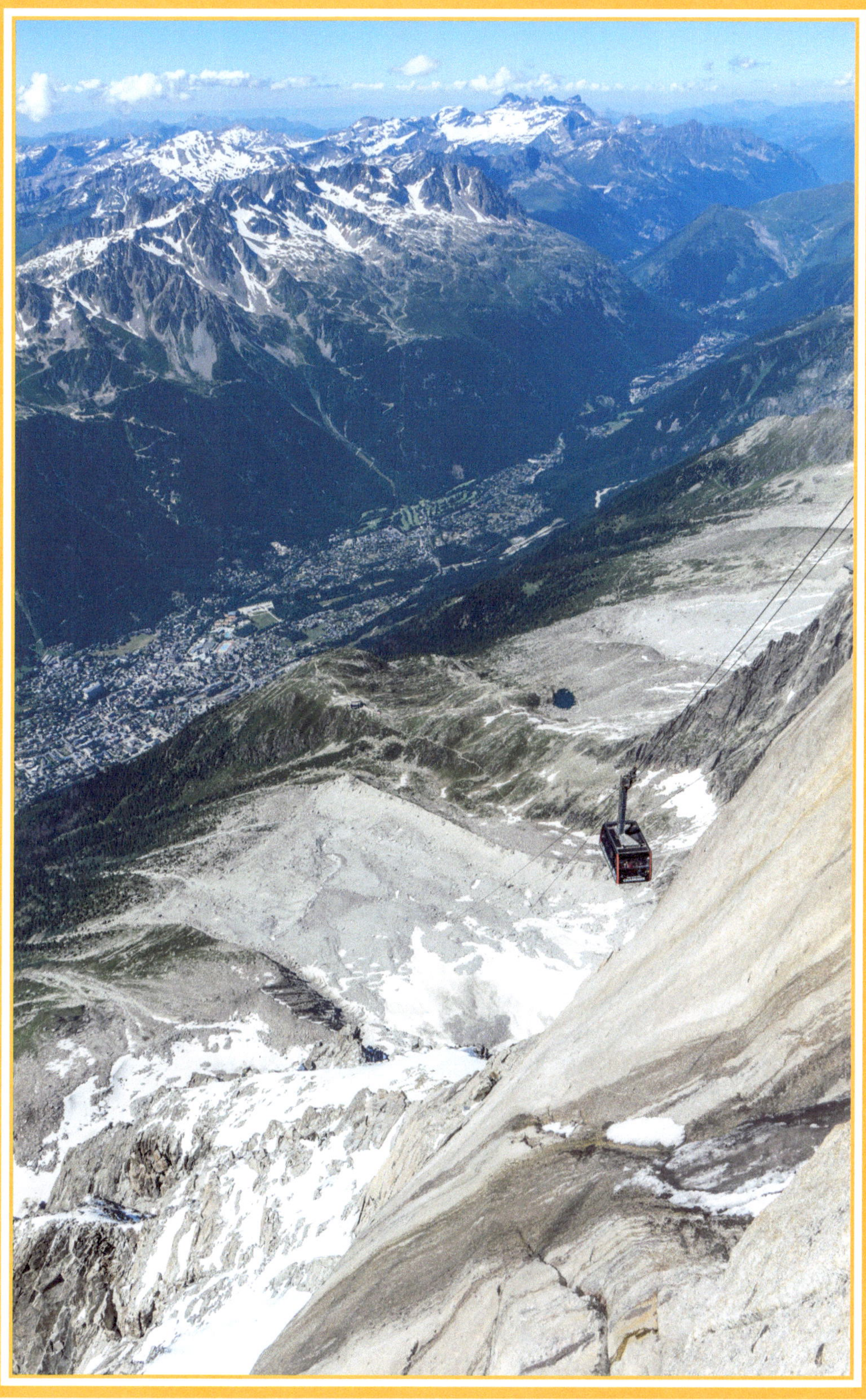

O praise the LORD,
all ye nations: praise
him all ye people.

Psalm 117:1

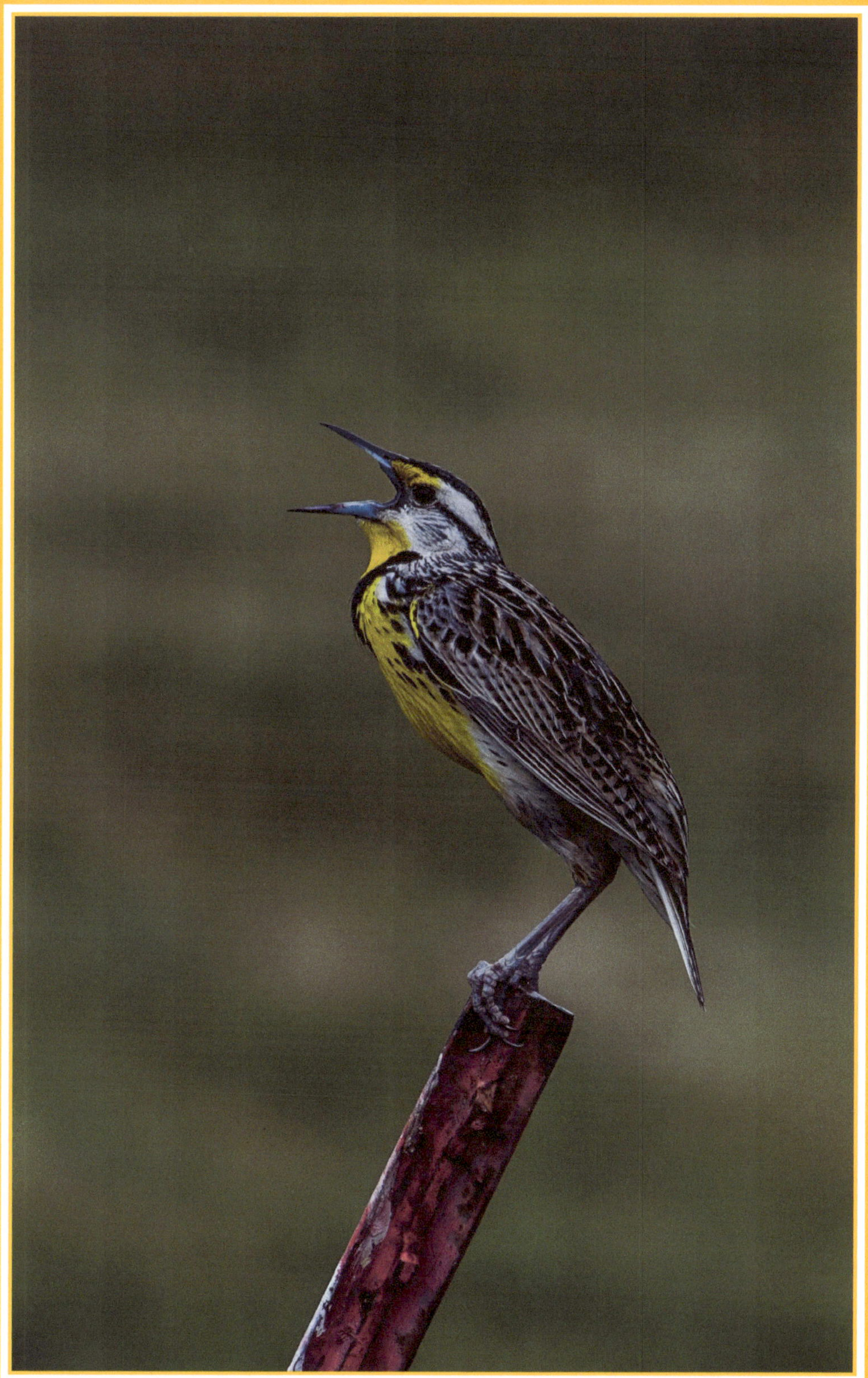

From the LORD
comes deliverance.
May your blessing
be on your people.

Psalm 3:8

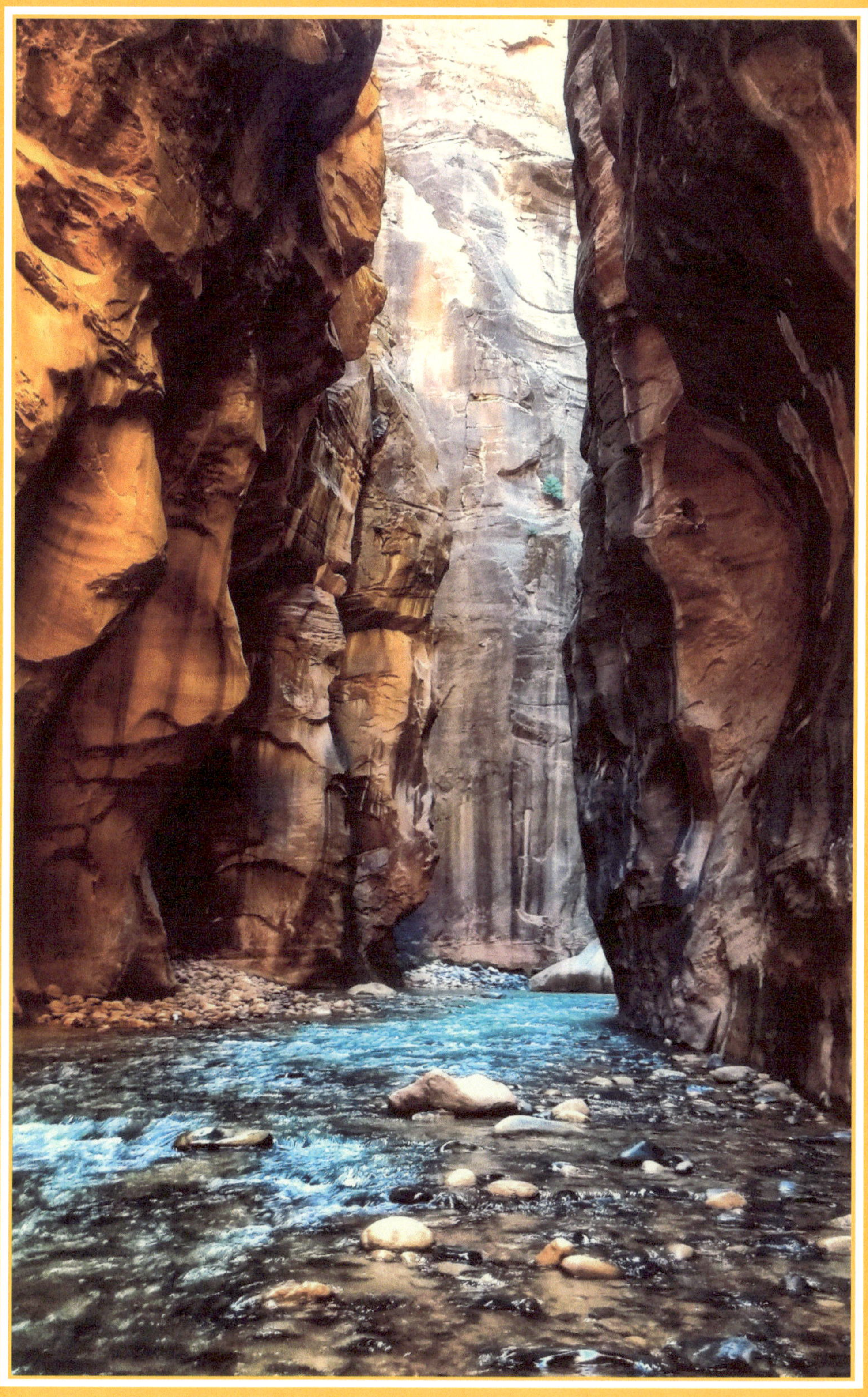

The LORD will keep
you from all harm—
he will watch over
your life.

Psalm 121:7

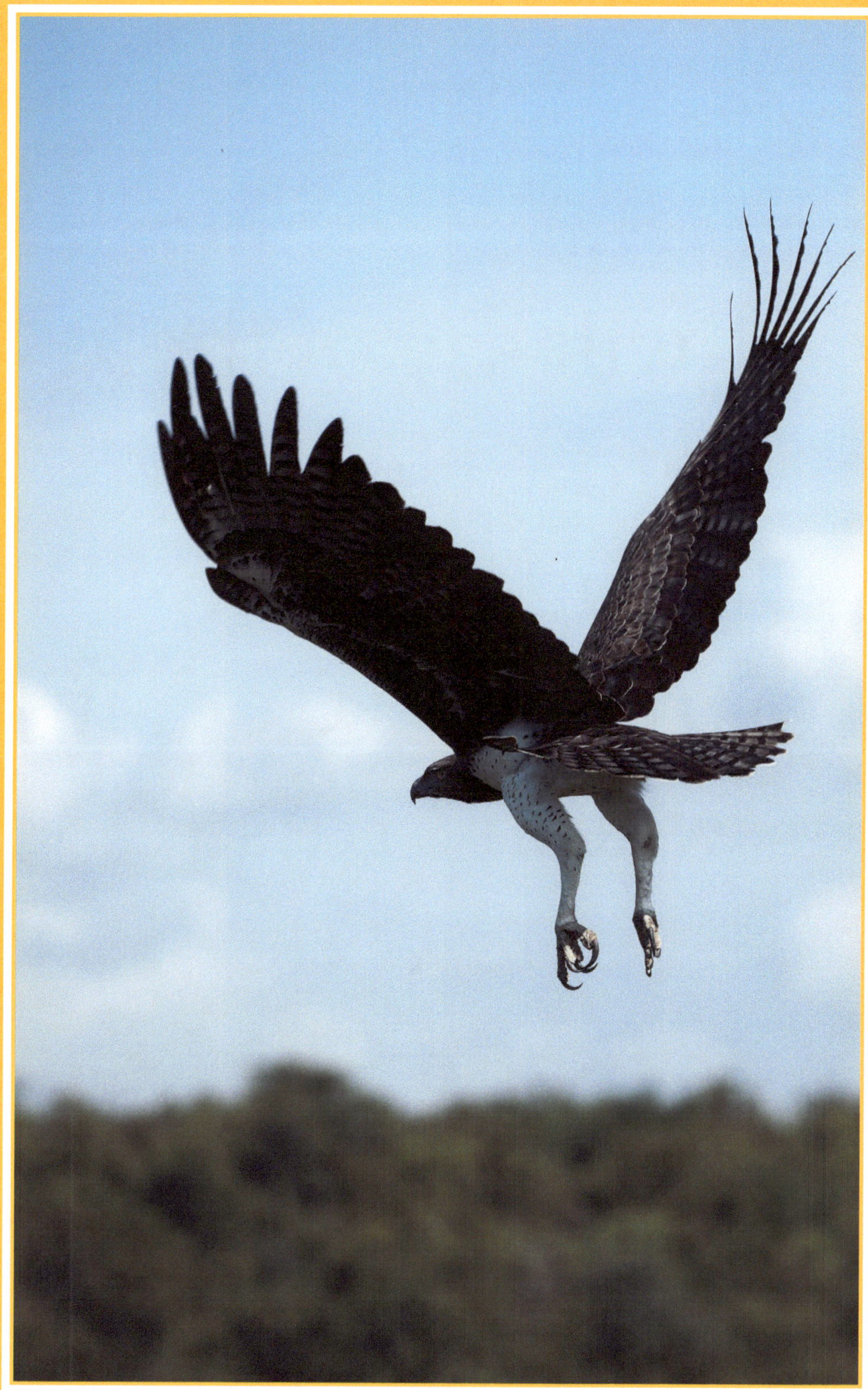

I will say of the Lord, "He is my refuge and my fortress, my God, in whom I trust."

Psalm 91:2

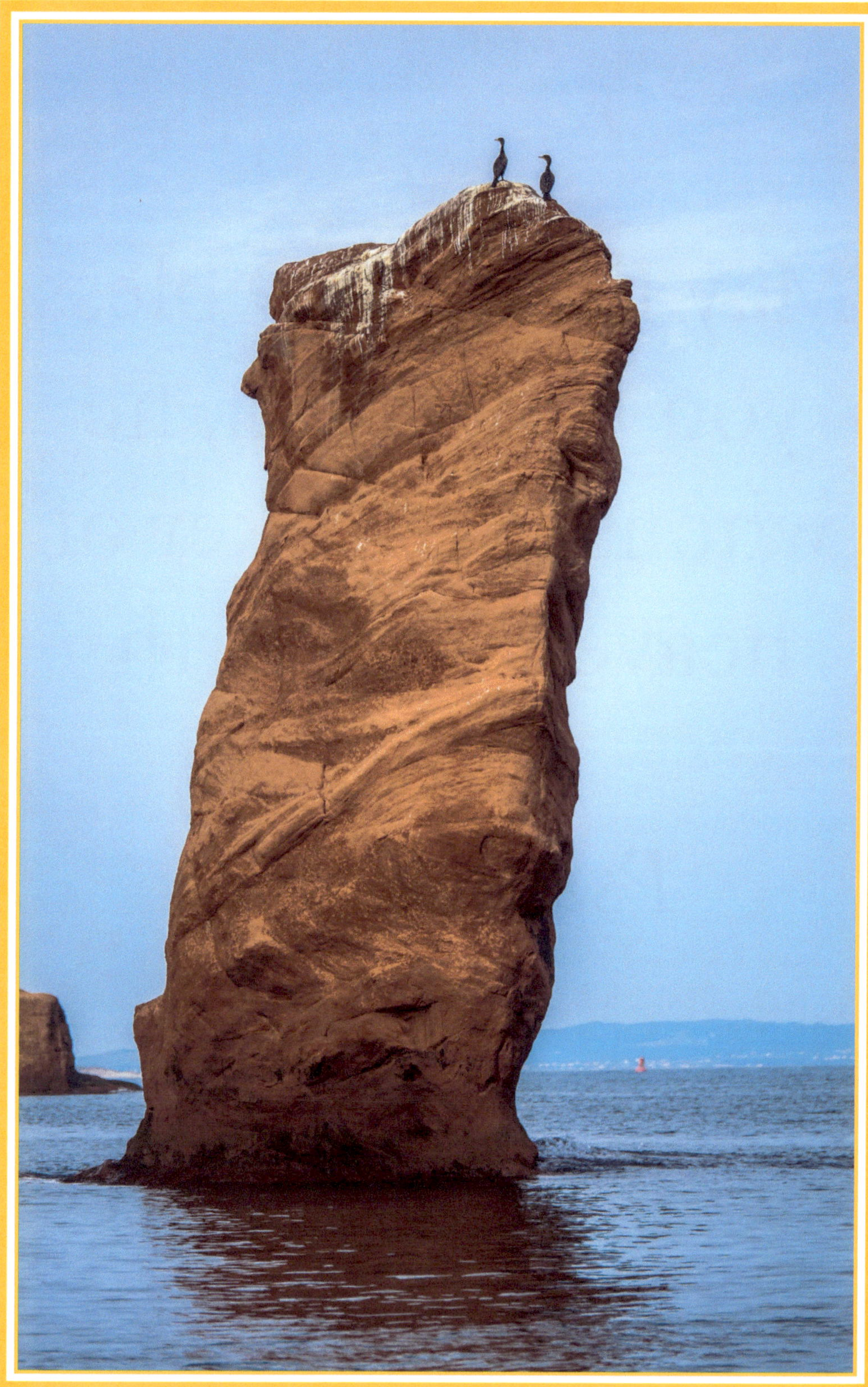

May the LORD bless you from Zion, he who is the Maker of heaven and earth.

Psalm 134:3

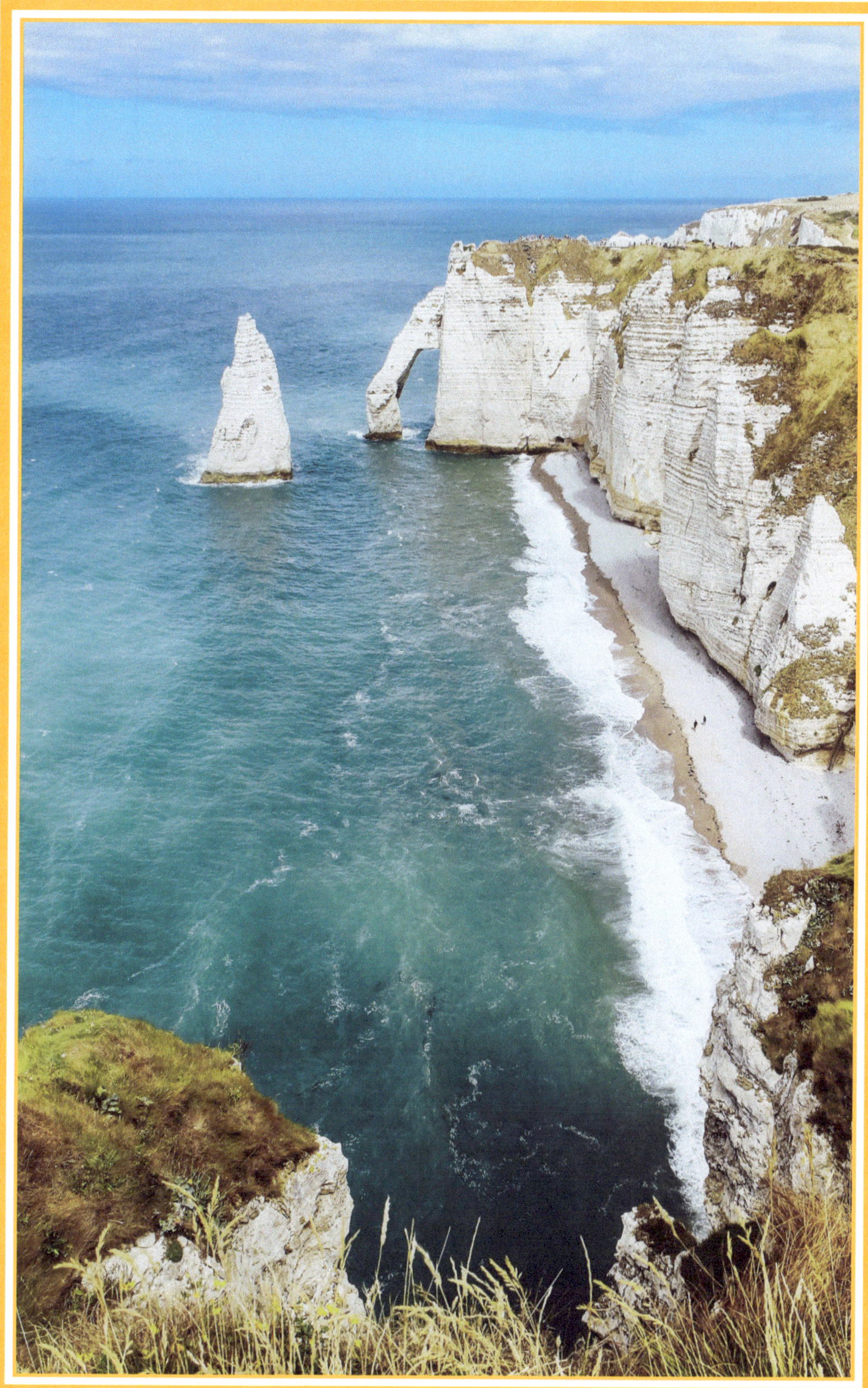

Hallelujah. Sing to the LORD a new song, his praise in the assembly of his faithful people.

Psalm 149:1

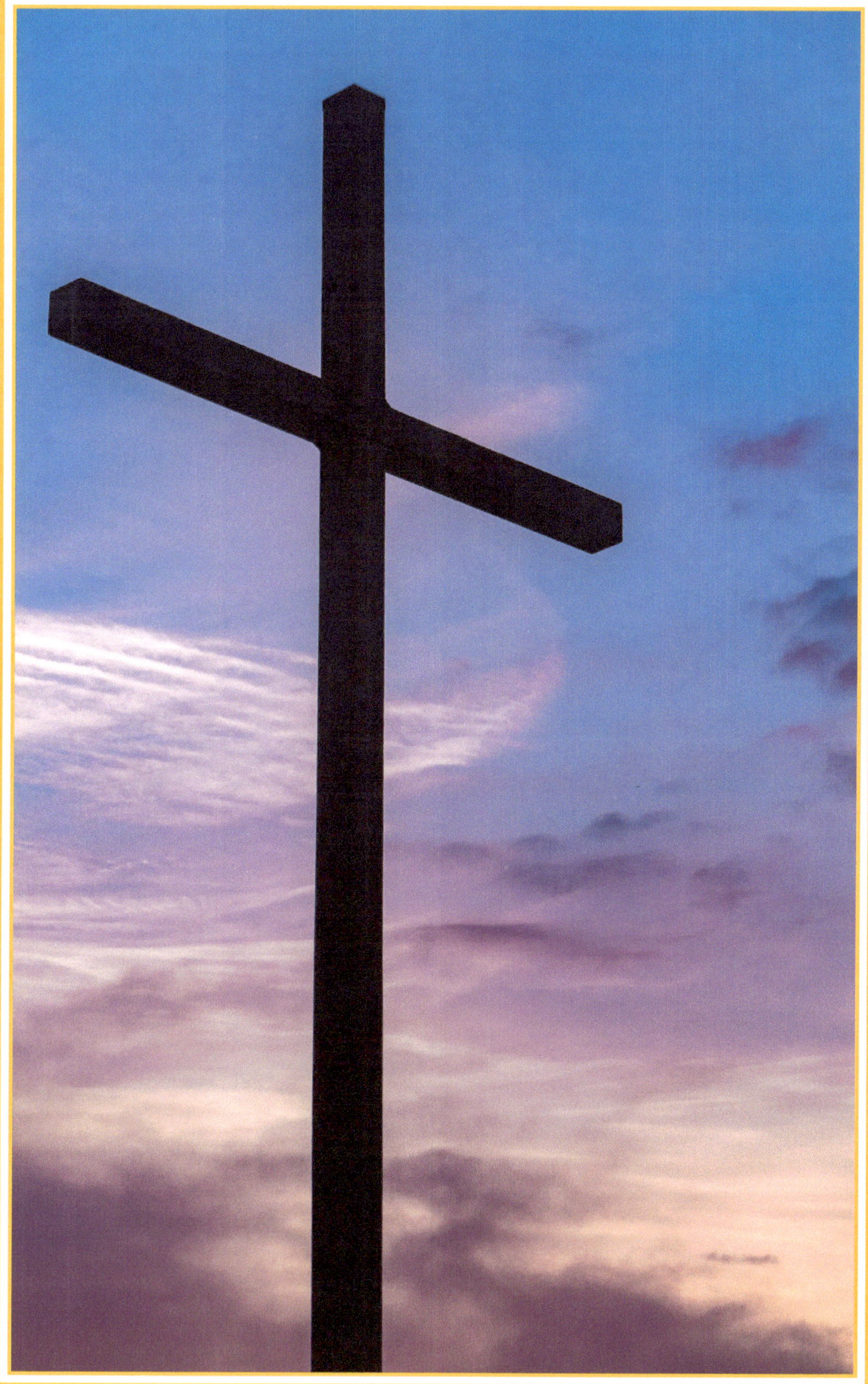

My shield is God
Most High, who
saves the upright
in heart.

Psalm 7:10

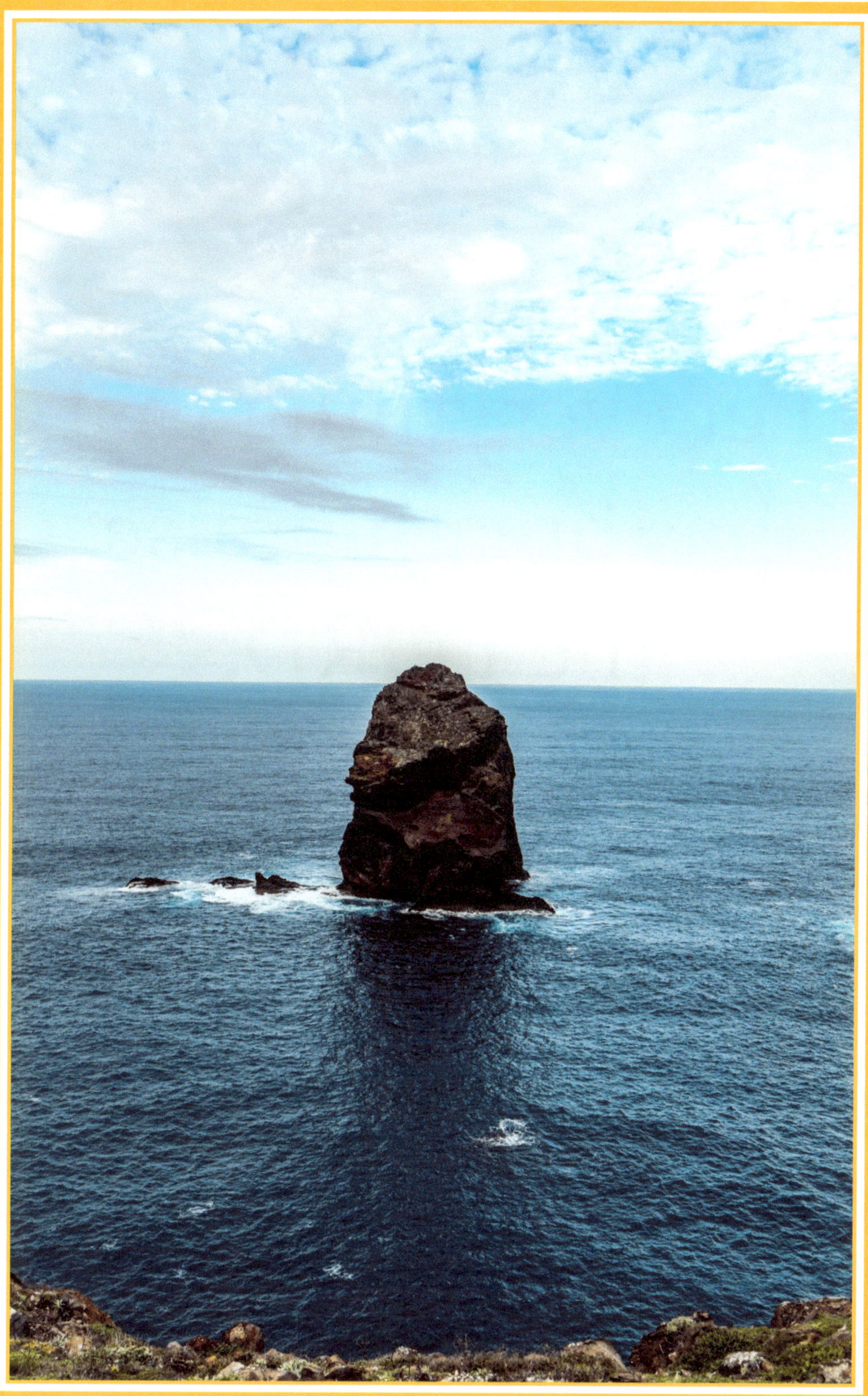

Let everything that
has breath praise
the LORD.

Psalm 150:6

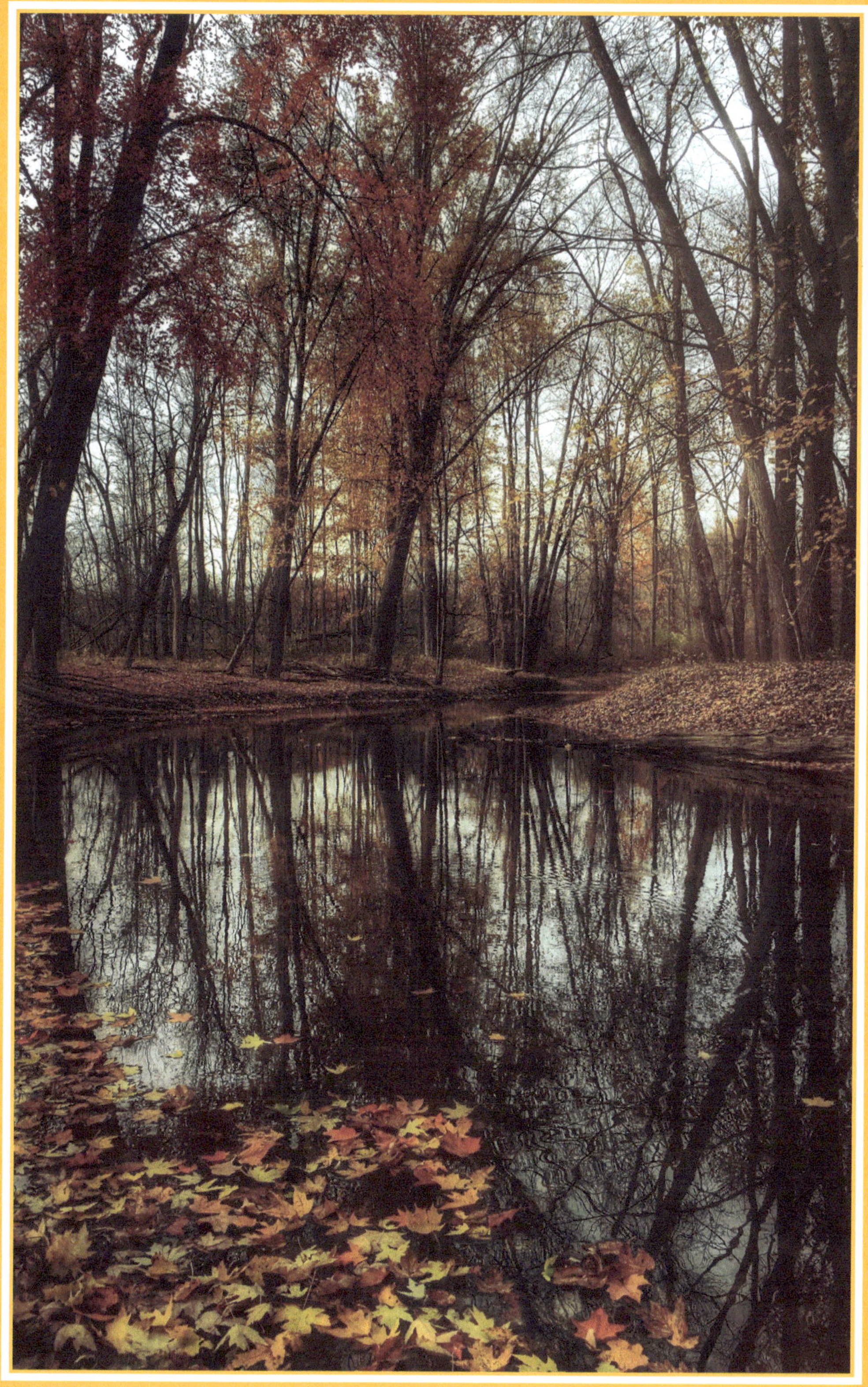

I call out to the
LORD, and he
answers me from
his holy mountain.

Psalm 3:4

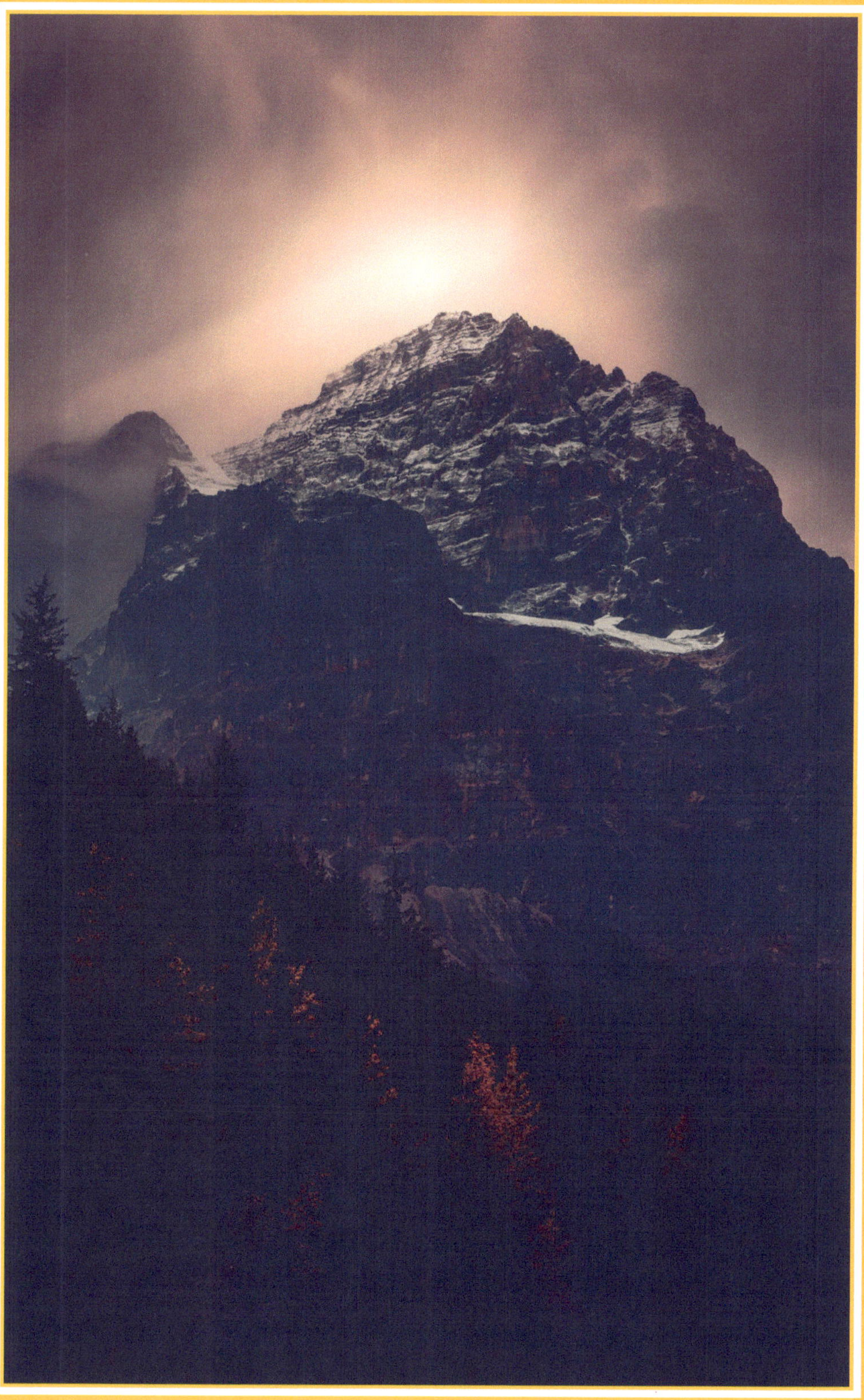

Surely, LORD, you bless the righteous; you surround them with your favor as with a shield.

Psalm 5:12

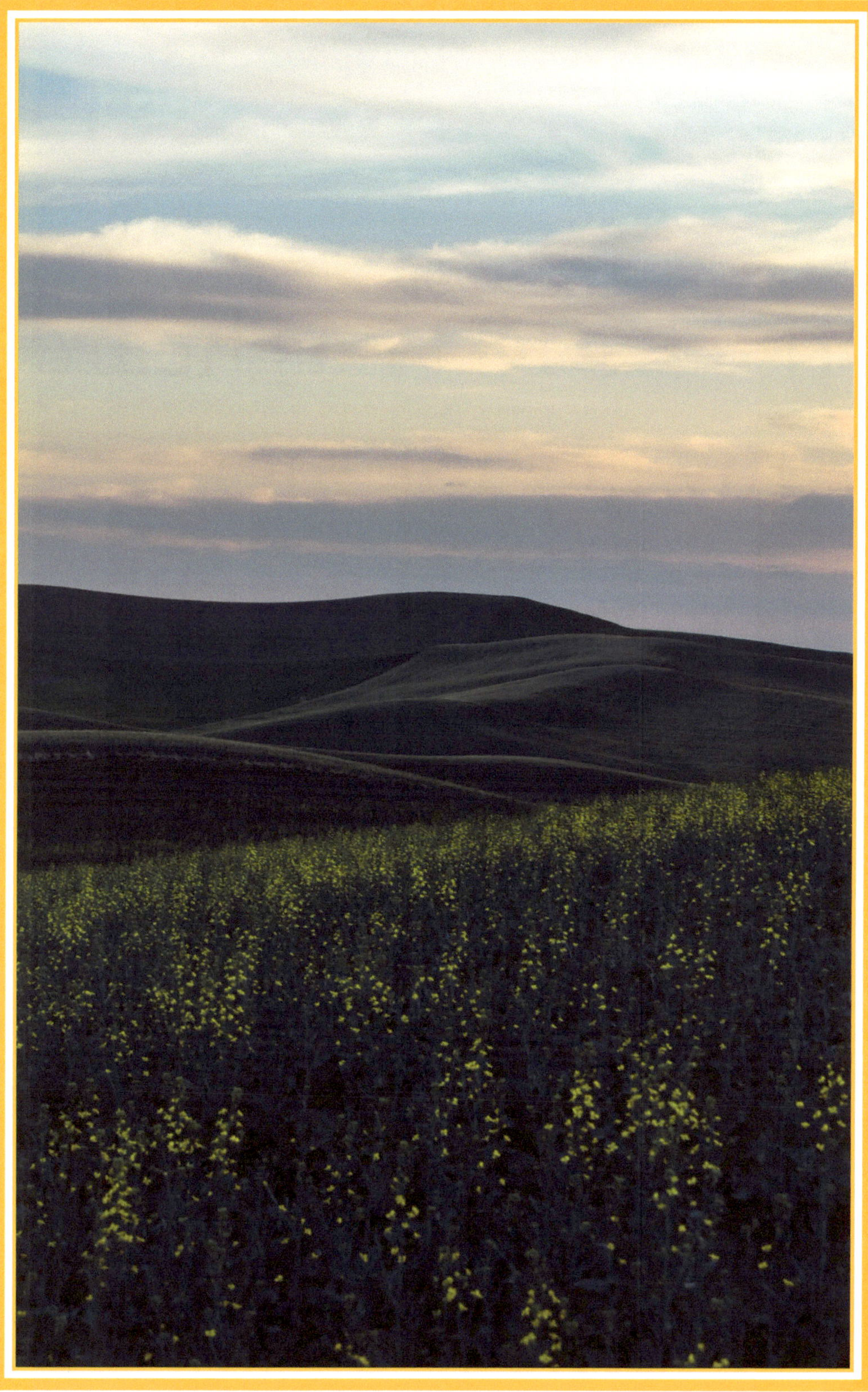

The LORD has heard my cry for mercy; the LORD accepts my prayer.

Psalm 6:9

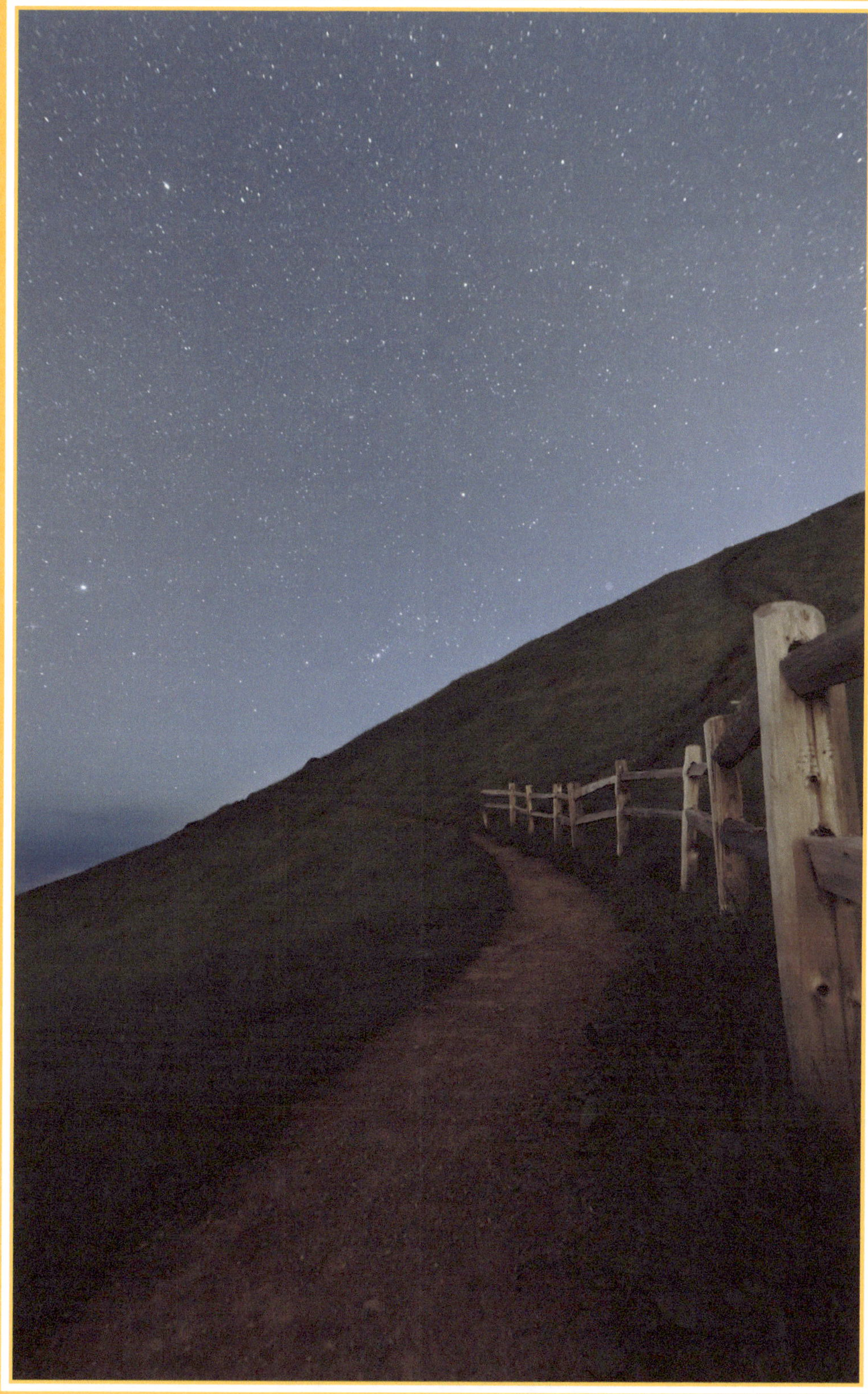